T0271947

REHABILITATION

FOR THE

UNWANTED

REHABILITATION
FOR THE
UNWANTED

PATIENTS AND THEIR CARETAKERS

JULIUS A. ROTH AND
ELIZABETH M. EDDY

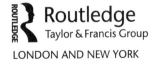 Routledge
Taylor & Francis Group

LONDON AND NEW YORK

First published 1967 by Transaction Publishers

Published 2017 by Routledge
2 Park Square, Milton Park, Abingdon, Oxon OX14 4RN
711 Third Avenue, New York, NY 10017, USA

Routledge is an imprint of the Taylor & Francis Group, an informa business

Library of Congress Catalog Number: 2010003494

Library of Congress Cataloging-in-Publication Data

Roth, Julius A.
  Rehabilitation for the unwanted : patients and their caretakers / Julius A. Roth and Elizabeth M. Eddy.
      p. cm.
  Originally published: New York : Atherton Press, c1967.
  Includes bibliographical references.
  ISBN 978-0-202-36352-3
    1. People with disabilities--Rehabilitation--United States.
  I. Eddy, Elizabeth M. II. Title.
RM930.R67 2010
362.3'3--dc22

                                                        2010003494

ISBN 13: 978-0-202-36352-3 (pbk)

Contents

Preface

By the time we were going through our fourth or fifth revision of this book we began to wish that we could write it in Chinese and thus escape the frustrating problem of verb tense. We could have written it as if it had all taken place in the past—and of course our observations *were* made in the past. But sometimes events can be more effectively presented as if they are going on in the present. Then there are still other occasions when we prefer to write as if our views and descriptions are timeless.

The last approach is the greatest fraud of all if taken literally. Our study must necessarily treat Farewell Hospital and its rehabilitation program in a moment of history—a "moment" in this case spread over nearly two years. We solved our verb tense problem (if "solved" can be used for a fabric of compromises) by using whatever tense struck us as making the most literary sense in a given passage. But we (and the reader) must take care not to forget that Farewell Hospital and "rehab" were constantly changing during those two years and have continued to change since we left.

But the issues which the hospital continues to face are likely to be similar and the manner of dealing with those issues which people think appropriate often will be the same as approaches used in the past. The question of what to do with, to, or for the rejects of our society becomes increasingly urgent. Despite the variations in detail of answering this question, basic lines of approach and development can be teased out—lines which will be repeated at different places and different times. It is with such an expectation in mind that we feel justified in regarding our book as more than a narrow slice of history.

We have thought it best for wider publication to keep the locale of our study anonymous. Therefore, all names in the text are fictitious, including Farewell Hospital. This name, by the way, is not just a wild fancy of ours; it was suggested by some patients who had a realistic view of what incarceration in this institution meant to them.

One unfortunate aspect of maintaining anonymity is the fact that we cannot acknowledge the help of the people who provided us with clearance and the many who served as our involuntary subjects. All these people at the very least tolerated our presence, which is all a professional snooper can reasonably ask for. Some of them went much farther and extended their friendship and shared their ideas on matters of common interest. Perhaps we will sometime be in a better position to thank them publicly by name.

We can, at any rate, give credit to those who helped us directly in our research and writing. Most important of all are the four—then graduate students—who carried out a substantial part of the field work during the most intensive part of the study: Edwin Chin Shong, G. Alexander Moore, Harry Slan, and Carl Wells. Chin Shong and Moore also read the early draft of our manuscript and made important changes and additions. Eliot Freidson, editor of this series, made suggestions which led to considerable reorganization and rewriting. Others who have read versions of the book at various stages and made suggestions ranging from new ways of looking at our materials to improving the readability of the copy include: Howard S. Becker, Robert Sommer, Dorothy J. Douglas, Pamela Landberg, and Jessica Roth. Because both authors have changed jobs and location since the study ended, the manuscript and the materials which preceded it have passed through a number of typists. We must give special mention, however, to the one who labored longest and most skillfully on doing our dirty work: Misako Mae Kanazawa.

And last, but not least, we must mention the source of funds which made the study possible: Research Grant No. RD-577 from the Vocational Rehabilitation Administration.

Rehabilitation for the unwanted

The end of the road   1

This book is about people who are at the end of the road, and what happens to them in a rehabilitation program, which implies that they have a future ahead of them. The program is embedded in an institution which exists to serve the demand that *some* kind of provision be made for those medical and social rejects who are judged unable to live on their own and who have no family or friends or other social agents who are willing to make a home for them outside of a public institution.

The rehabilitation program we observed failed to alter significantly the careers of most of these patients. The most important learning for the patients was not the physical techniques which might enable them to return to meaningful lives in the community. Rather, they learned that they were too incapacitated to gain much from the rehabilitation program, or even if they succeeded in markedly improving their physical abilities, that they had no one or no place on the outside willing to receive a still partially disabled person. Most patients learned that placement on the rehabilitation unit was just a brief interlude before more permanent placement in a custodial unit in the vast institution which we call Farewell Hospital, where they would live out their lives.

Although our study focuses on a physical rehabilitation program, we cannot help but constantly take into account the great complex of buildings and people of which this program is only a small part. Farewell Hospital is in the middle of a large city, but is isolated. Its staff roster lists numerous and various members of "helping" occupations, but the inmates are largely left to their fate. The hospital has a reputation as a repository for the city's unwanted disabled people.

In this unpromising setting, "rehab" tries to come to the rescue. Despite the non-therapeutic (often anti-therapeutic) rules and practices of the larger health and welfare structure of which they are a part, the rehab specialists and ward workers set themselves the task of improving the life chances of their involuntary clients by treating their ailments when possible and by improving their physical functioning so that they will be better able to care for their own needs. With their far-from-ideal patients—mostly aged with disabling chronic diseases and without interested families—their accomplishments *by their own standards* are very limited, in many cases nil.

In examining this program which, more often than not, failed to accomplish its goal, we will be concerned not simply with the characteristics of the staff and the patients and the details of the therapy programs. Rather, we will focus on the organization of relationships within the institutional setting—a setting which itself is a product of and reaction to the larger society. We will examine the effects of the organizational relationships on the rehabilitation outcomes and on the lives of the people who make Farewell Hospital their home. We will also attempt to sustain some feeling for the historical context of our study—the "problem" of larger and larger numbers of disabled, poverty-stricken persons, who are no longer wanted by anyone and for whom a "solution" must be found.

Background to rehab

Rehabilitation medicine is a relatively new medical specialty. Although many of the concepts and some of the techniques can no doubt be traced back for decades and even centuries, the specialty received its greatest impetus during and immediately after World War II when there was an obvious moral mandate to give all possible assistance to the large number of youthful disabled veterans in their effort to return to some degree of physical "normality." After the crest of this war-damaged population had passed through the hospitals, this growing specialty needed to find new reasons for its existence.*

Rehabilitation medicine now began to define itself as a salvage operation—not curing disease or repairing injury, but restoring, at least partially, physical capacities after the damage had been done. Rehabilitation medicine, in fact, took a road common to newly developing occupations—staking out a territory which is not yet occupied. Thus, resistance from established occupations (or specialties) is at a minimum and the opportunity to experiment with new approaches is at a maximum. Of course, the new approaches and diversification of

* For a more detailed history of the rehabilitation movement see Robert Straus, "Social Change and the Rehabilitation Concept," in *Sociology and Rehabilitation,* Marvin Sussman, ed., American Sociological Association. (No date.) Recently, leading medical institutions have begun to change the title of departments, formerly known as Departments of Physical Medicine and Rehabilitation, to Departments of Rehabilitation Medicine. This is but one indication of the attempt of physiatrists to define their own new medical specialty.

tasks eventually tread across the boundaries of an established discipline, but by that time the newer group may be well enough accepted to hold its own in the jurisdictional dispute.

Rehabilitation medicine thus began to take on the patients which other branches of medicine tended to ignore. Rehab specialists concerned themselves with the physical functioning and retraining of the traumatically injured after the surgeon had done his work. Even more significantly, they took on the care and rehabilitation of persons with incurable skeletal, muscular, and neurological diseases and defects—a group which medicine traditionally tended to regard as hopeless and not worth wasting time and effort on. Not only did this "salvage operation" give rehabilitation physicians (physiatrists, as they are often called) a relatively unoccupied territory to work in, but it also gave them a cause to promote and thus earn their specialty greater attention from related occupations, from foundations and government granting agencies, and from the voting and taxpaying public. Much of the crusading spirit and enthusiasm which one can still note in rehabilitation staffs (in much of their workaday activities, not just their propaganda literature) stems from the feeling that they must overcome the inertia of the older medical specialties in order to obtain care and treatment of the neglected disabled.

Rehab self-consciously defines itself as a salvage operation. But within any given treatment context, some human beings are more salvageable than others. Programs purporting to help the poor, the jobless, the sick, the discriminated-against, and the otherwise stigmatized typically select for their clientele those who are judged to show most promise of a successful result within the framework of program facilities and programmatic definitions of success and failure. This process leaves a new residue of rejects who may in turn become the focus of attention of still another assistance program of lesser status.*

* See Martin Rein, "The Social Service Crisis," *Trans-action,* vol. I

The rehab program at Farewell Hospital is no exception to the effort to select the "cream" of the population of potential candidates. However, the population available to the rehab staff is for the most part in such poor physical condition as a result of serious chronic illness and advanced age that even the cream has mostly poor candidates for rehabilitation, a point which will be detailed in later chapters.

The rehab team

Rehabilitation medicine did not occupy its territory as an isolated discipline, but carried with it several supporting occupations. The one whose fate is most closely linked with rehabilitation medicine is physical therapy (PT). Although physical therapists do have career opportunities outside the physical rehabilitation field, a large portion of them (especially the women) work in rehab programs. Looking at it another way, rehab programs always employ PTs and, in the program we observed, they sometimes seemed more essential than the physicians in charge.

Occupational therapy, medical social work, speech and hearing therapy, and vocational rehabilitation counseling are less closely linked to physical rehabilitation programs, both because such programs sometimes get along without them and because rehab represents only a small proportion of the career opportunities open to these professional groups. Clinical psychologists, group workers, and recreation workers are even more tangentially related to rehab and are often regarded as frills which can be dispensed with readily.

The division of labor and the nature of the relationships between the professional specialties will be the subject of Chapter 5. We will give special attention to the work role of two subspecies of social workers to show how members of a profes-

(May 1964), pp. 3–6, 31–32, for a discussion of this selective process in social agencies.

sional group with aspirations toward autonomy fare in a rather rigid organization where their definition of their work role is not accepted by those who have authority over them.

The various rehab specialists in a given institution often refer to themselves as a "team." The physicians are expected to listen to the advice of the supporting professionals and give them more decision-making power than physicians traditionally give "paramedical" workers. The reader can judge from the chapter on the team the extent to which this concept is operational. The aspect which struck us, however, was that the group most directly and continuously involved in patient care—the ward staff—was not a part of this team. True, there was a nurse (usually the unit supervisor or head nurse) present at most team meetings, but this nurse typically took far less part in the discussions than anyone else. Other ward personnel had an even lesser role in team decisions. We will devote Chapter 4 to this important group, which serves as the whipping boy for both the patients and the other professional disciplines.

The clients

From the viewpoint of those patients selected for rehab, the rehab wards are not simply a treatment locale, but a home— sometimes for an extended period. It is a home in which they are involuntarily crowded in with others who may be somewhat similar in their physical disabilities, but often dissimilar in other respects. They construct a small society which in some respects resembles the larger society from which they came.

To the patients the rehab program may at first seem like another chance to learn to get about and to care for themselves and eventually escape from the institution. They soon find, however, that the rehab wards are not designed to meet many of their daily needs, and the more helpless they are, the greater their difficulty in getting their wants taken care of, a point made in Chapter 3 with regard to mobility and other physical activities.

As an institutional inmate, the patient must make decisions about how he is going to cope with the social structure in which he has been placed—a structure in whose development he had no part, but to which he is expected to "adapt." Chapter 7 describes some typical coping patterns which we observed among the inmates and Chapter 8 relates some of the ways in which inmates create areas of choice in the interstices of the "system." Both chapters draw heavily on Erving Goffman's analysis of total institutions.*

The inmates find too that the workings of the bureaucratic health and welfare structure in which they have been deposited have severely limited their future alternatives and their chances of ever again living outside an institution. The very slowness with which the wheels turn cause them to lose their homes and their financial assets, dissipate relationships with people who might earlier have helped them, and allow them to become adapted to institutional living as an easier alternative to the struggle to get out. Enforced indigency, unavailability of housing for persons not able to fend for themselves, failure of hospital personnel to consult patients about decisions affecting their own lives, all contribute to subverting the announced goals of the rehab program and turning most patients into permanent inmates. These points are documented in Chapters 6, 9, and 10.

In Chapter 10 we will also examine explicitly some of the outcomes of the rehab program. We will use the staff's own working definitions of success and failure to measure how they fared. We will present evidence to support our assertion that the program was largely a failure from the point of view of both the staff and the patients.

* Erving Goffman, *Asylums* (Garden City, N.Y.: Doubleday, 1961). See especially the essay entitled "On the Characteristics of Total Institutions," pp. 12–60.

The institutional setting

Rehabilitation medicine is almost entirely "institutional medicine." Even private patients who are living at home typically come to a hospital rather than to a physician's office for treatment and evaluation. Rehabilitation is also frequently organized into programs involving numerous patients rather than consisting of treating a series of individuals. Thus, the study of the rehabilitation process will usually involve the study of an institutional setting.

Our study includes only one rehab program in one large public chronic-disease hospital. Our acquaintance with descriptions of other large institutions with programs of treatment for people in various states and degrees of helplessness leads us to believe that the program and the setting we observed are not unique. It is simply one of the more striking examples of the disposition of the disabled rejects of our modern urban society. Similar depositories for rejects with a variety of labels and ostensible purposes already exist and are likely to become more common. The creation of such institutions will probably be accelerated by Medicare, which provides a convenient "solution" for families and welfare agencies to dispose of the burdensome aged, largely at federal expense. Special programs of assistance may make the life of such social rejects a little more tolerable and will even rescue a few of them, but unless we pay more attention to the organizational structure in which such programs are carried out and the nature of the alternatives provided the client population, the efforts of these programs may be largely dissipated and even subverted. Our final chapter will comment on some of the issues raised by the institutional treatment of people whose chief disability is that they are unwanted.

The rehab clientele and its selection 2

In one twelve-month period during the time of this study about 850 persons were discharged from Farewell Hospital. Almost two-thirds of them were dead. It is literally a place where people are sent to die. For the most part, they do not die quickly. The turnover is slow indeed for a place that calls itself a hospital. The nearly 2,000 beds are almost all filled, yet there are only about 800 admissions and a like number of discharges a year.

Most of the patients have had long periods of hospitalization for chronic illness or physical defects before coming to Farewell. There was a point at which physicians in a general hospital, usually also a public hospital in the same city, decided there was no likelihood of a cure or substantial improvement. The patient was taking up space in an acute treatment unit and had to be moved out. If he was judged not able to get along completely on his own and if he did not have a family or friends willing and able to provide for him, he was a prime candidate for custodial care—"the prolonged hospitalization of the type Farewell affords"—as one referring physician bluntly put it in his final discharge notes.

Such are the patients Farewell typically receives. Most are aged, poverty-stricken, chronically ill, and within a few years of death. Typically, they have a variety of physical ailments. Some are totally bedridden; others are ambulatory and take care of their own bodily needs; most are between these poles.

Almost all are receiving public assistance of some sort when they arrive, or must go on the assistance rolls not long thereafter when their assets have been consumed. (We found some of these patients denying that they had ever received "welfare," not realizing that their current hospital expenses were being met by the local welfare department.) In some cases, the family and friends of the patient cannot be traced. When traced, many show no interest in offering the patient a home.

With few exceptions, these patients have not been consulted about their removal to Farewell Hospital. Some arrive there not knowing where they are or why they have been moved. They have been "dumped." In fact, Farewell is openly referred to by some of the staff as the dumping ground of the city hospital system.

Selection for rehabilitation

In this unpromising setting, the rehab staff tries to inject some hope and promise. These medical and social rejects should not be allowed to "rot away" on the hospital's back wards. With

expert treatment, exercises, retraining, and properly fitted
prostheses and assistive appliances, the patient with "motivation" can be improved to a point where he can get about by
himself, care for his own needs, even live outside an institution. Of course, this program cannot be offered to all patients
entering Farewell Hospital. Rehab has only one hundred beds
on its active unit, another one hundred on a nursing unit
without the rehab team program (in fact, we found on close
examination, no program at all). Then, too, some patients are
judged poor candidates for rehab—that is, the patient's condition is such that he seems unlikely to benefit from the treatment rehab has to offer. This means that a selection must be
made from the available pool of patients.

The selection of about half of all the patients taken on the
active rehab unit is carried out in a weekly line-up where
the rehab director or one of his senior physicians looks over the
patients who were admitted to Farewell Hospital during the
previous week or so. The physician allows himself about one
hour to evaluate twelve to fifteen patients whose person and
records he is seeing for the first time. Most of the patients are
completely unaware of the nature of the clinic or the crucial
importance it has for their future placement. As they walk
up, or more often are pushed up in a wheelchair, to the physician's table, they are asked a few questions about the nature
of their disability. Sometimes the questions are intended only
to test the patient's mental orientation and any confusion or
lack of fluency on his part is likely to be held against him.
The questioning is so superficial that it occasionally fails to
discover that the patient's lack of response is the result of
speaking only a foreign language.

If the patient looks like a possibility, he may be asked to perform briefly (e.g., stand, walk). The physician will also skim
the patient's records. ("Read" does not seem the correct word
for the rapid flipping of pages observed in most cases.) The
physician then renders a decision. The patient may be assigned
to the active rehab program, as were 12 out of 119 in eleven

clinics observed. He may be assigned to the inactive rehab nursing unit (6 out of 119). He may be scheduled for the nursing self-care program, a limited program for non-rehab patients intended to retrain patients in self-care activities (37 out of 119). Or no recommendation may be made, leaving the patient's placement to other physicians, but rejecting him from rehab for the time being at least (64 out of 119).

To be selected for rehab, the patient must have the "right" disability. Almost all those taken on rehab during our study had hemiplegia (lateral paralysis in most cases resulting from cerebral vascular occlusion or rupture of a blood vessel—commonly called a "stroke"), amputation of one or both legs, spinal cord injury resulting in partial paralysis, multiple sclerosis, arthritis, muscular dystrophy, or an improperly healed fracture. Having the right disability was not enough, however. Of the 119 patients observed in the selection process, 33 had disabilities in the appropriate categories but were rejected. Age is a factor: the rehab staff has a strong bias in favor of youth, a bias difficult to implement in this largely aged population. Those chosen for the active and inactive rehab wards averaged sixty-seven years old (half were sixty or less); those rejected averaged seventy-three (80 percent over sixty). Simply being below fifty and having the right kind of disability almost guaranteed selection for rehab.

The sheer weight given to youth was most dramatically illustrated in the case of a twenty-year-old quadriplegic who appeared at a selection clinic. He had already been under treatment for two years in other hospitals with no noticeable improvement. The physician sought excuses to avoid consigning him to the back wards with the aged "vegetables." He even asked the patient loaded questions and dropped hints about what the right answers were. But the apathetic patient missed his cues and gave responses which made him appear hopeless. Despite the discouraging picture, the doctor compromised by assigning him to the rehab nursing unit, and within a month, at the recommendation of the physical therapists, he transferred him to the active program. Here the patient received a grossly disproportionate amount of the therapists' time, again without noticeable improvement.

The over-all principle of selection is that the patient should be amenable to help from rehab training and activities. If his over-all physical condition is severely deteriorated, he is less likely to benefit from the program and therefore he is more likely to be rejected. On the other hand, if he is able to take physical care of himself without assistance (and a few such cases *do* show up), he does not *need* rehab. Thus, the rehab candidate should not be in too good or too bad a shape. He should show sufficient mental alertness to be judged capable of learning the therapeutic teachings. And he should not be so apathetic as to be judged completely lacking in "motivation" to improve—a vague but important concept about which we will have more to say.

Other routes to rehab

The selection clinic is not the patient's only chance at getting on rehab. Physicians on other services sometimes refer promising cases to rehab for consultation. Other patients are sent to the prosthetic clinic run by the rehab staff to obtain a prescription for an apparently needed prosthesis or appliance. Some of these referrals make a good impression on the rehab physicians and are transferred to the active rehab program. A patient who appears mentally dull at the initial selection (perhaps because of a recent stroke) may recover spontaneously in a month or two, to the point where he seems to be a good prospect to relearn the use of his paralyzed limbs. About one-fourth of the rehab patients entered the program through intra-hospital referral during our period of observation.

While the selection of some patients is delayed, others are preselected. The same physicians who work on the rehab program also are on the staff of a public general hospital. At times they find patients in the general hospital who are unlikely to recover in the near future, but who are judged to have the potential for significant improvement in a long-term retraining program. Such patients may then be transferred directly from the general hospital to the Farewell rehab ward.

Almost all patients entered rehab through one of these three routes at the time of this study. A few others were accepted after referral by outside physicians, special pleading by a patient's family or influential acquaintance, or as a part of the rehabilitation service's participation in a special program.

Patient participation in selection

Farewell Hospital is not likely to be chosen by many people as a place of retirement. But according to common opinion among those who know the place, if you *must* stay at Farewell, you are better off on rehab than anywhere else. It has a larger complement of professional personnel interested in the patients; it has more younger patients and fewer grossly deteriorated, vegetable-like patients (and consequently is less odoriferous); it offers more recreational activities (often disguised as therapy); and for those who still have hope of improvement in their physical condition, rehab holds out the most hope. Then too, in some circles outside the hospital, the Farewell rehab unit has a reputation for specializing in the treatment of certain disorders (e.g., arthritis, muscular dystrophy), and patients with these conditions or persons interested in their welfare may make an effort to obtain admission to the rehab program.

In most cases, patients have no part in selection decisions. Within Farewell, patients who appear at the selection clinic usually do not know why they are there, and when they are questioned a short time afterward, most are not aware that important decisions have been made about them. Similarly, those who arrive on rehab as a result of direct transfer from other wards or hospitals do not have any specific idea of where they are or that they are to begin or continue a program of rehabilitation. This lack of knowledge on the part of most patients does not vary systematically with the disability, age, education, or socioeconomic background of the patients, but is rather related to their subordinate status and the fact that they are not defined as those who must or should be fully informed about what is happening to them.

A small proportion of patients are better informed. These patients have heard about the rehab wards at Farewell. When their hospital insurance has been exhausted and bed space at their previous hospitals is no longer available for this or other reasons, they are told of "the better care and therapy at Farewell." One patient, for example, was specifically told that rehab at Farewell is "the big thing" and explained that she would have come earlier if space had been available. Another had heard "raves about Farewell," and one of the health foundations had recommended she come.

Patients may not only act on their own behalf but they may also have agents who act on their behalf. Letters about patients are infrequent, but physicians, social workers, hospital administrators, and the clergy occasionally write them and may even specifically request that the patient be placed on rehab. Five patients directly transferred to the rehab wards from voluntary private and public hospitals—which were unconnected with the medical center of which Farewell is a part—had also been specifically told about the rehab program at Farewell and arrived with the definite expectation of receiving therapy which would substantially aid them. Of these, four were directly transferred to rehab as a result of letters to the director of the rehab service or the medical director at Farewell. In one case, the son of an aphasic was able to answer the physician's questions at the selection clinic and attracted attention to his father's case.

In general, the patients who are informed about the rehab wards and have the capacity to act as their own agents or to have others act on their behalf are apt to be selected for rehab. At the selection clinic, they are in a position to present their desires and almost invariably do so. Nearly always, they are chosen even though the physician may feel that little can be done to help them and may only take them to prevent their "rotting away" on the less desirable wards.

Our study cases

Our study of the Farewell rehab wards was focused initially on the way in which the patients cope with their life situation. This meant collecting information about the world which most immediately affected the patients—their fellow inmates around the institution, the organization, decision-making, and work practices of the staff, the role of the larger health and welfare system and outside organizations. We spent much time in the hospital, mostly on rehab, seeing what took place at various times on the wards, the therapy areas, the hallways. We attended staff meetings, especially those concerned with decisions about patients. We talked to patients and staff about hospital life and various aspects of the program. We read patient records and rehab literature.*

As we came to identify the issues which were important to the people in the hospital and made plans to keep more detailed records of our observations, it seemed that it would be useful to have a series of thoroughly studied patient careers to draw on for the following purposes:

1. Make frequency statements about a group of patients for whom we had comprehensive, fairly accurate, and comparable information.

2. Reconstruct typical career patterns with longitudinal data rather than having to rely solely on records and someone's memory.

* For more details on our data-gathering, see Appendix A.

3. Provide a context for interpreting patients' behavior in particular crucial incidents.

4. Provide a context for interpreting staff decisions concerning patients.

We did not want only "typical" patients, but all the kinds which rehab dealt with—the unusual or extreme cases are often the most instructive. We therefore decided to include all successive admissions to the active rehab wards for a period of time—sixty patients over a period of about five months, as it turned out. We followed their cases closely and intensively throughout their stay on the rehab wards, though three of them were still there when we finally retired from the scene about a year and a half later, and for those who remained in Farewell we made one or more follow-up visits after they were transferred off rehab. It is these sixty patients whom we will frequently refer to in this book with such phrases as "our special sample" or "our sample of sixty."

Half of our sample of sixty are over sixty years old while 80 percent of all Farewell admissions are over sixty. In our sample, 60 percent have an occupational background of semi-skilled or unskilled labor or no occupation at all; another 22 percent have "clerical and sales" background, but usually of a very low level; 51 percent of the males and 83 percent of the females are single, widowed, separated, or divorced (to say nothing of the virtually separated status of some of those still officially married). Of these patients, 35 percent have no family or interested friends at all at the time of hospitalization; 15 percent have some family in the area, but the family shows no interest whatever in their welfare; another 15 percent initially had an interested family, but the family lost interest during their period of hospitalization.

The largest disability group in our special sample are the hemiplegics, with amputees and multiple sclerosis victims next in order. There were only two spinal cord injuries in our sample, though quadriplegics and paraplegics form a much larger proportion of the ward population because they tend to stay much longer than other disability groups.*

Such "vital statistics" help set the stage. More important to an understanding of Farewell Hospital and its rehab program, however, are the details of patients' activities and relationships and the manner in which these are evaluated and controlled by the rehab staff. The next several chapters are addressed to these issues. While we will be primarily concerned with our sample of sixty, we will also draw on observational material made on others with whom they lived and shared experiences during their stay on rehab.

---

* Appendix B contains tabulations of some social and disability characteristics of the sample of sixty.

Society in miniature 3

Just as in our larger society, the social rewards of Farewell patients are not distributed evenly, but depend on the patients' place in the "status system" and on their ability (or the ability of their agents) to exert control over those who serve them.

In general, the more severely disabled a patient is (and thus, the more help he "deserves"), the less he gets out of life in Farewell, including rehab. Among the activities available to patients, the selective influences of both staff and patients tend to keep patients from lower status categories out of higher status activities, and in many cases keep the lowly from *any* formally sponsored activity.

To document these points, we will first examine patients' patterns of activity.

The daily round

The casual visitor strolling through the wards of Farewell Hospital is likely to be left with an impression of massive inactivity. Large numbers of patients are lying or sitting around "doing nothing," often looking vacant and out of contact with the world. Much of the institution resembles the stereotype of the more primitive state mental hospitals.

The rehab unit shows the most activity of any ward in the hospital. But even here, when one visits the ward at a time between meals or in the evening when no special program is going on, most patients will seem more or less immobile and not much interested in their surroundings, including other people. This impression is in part misleading because the most active patients are likely to be off the ward out-of-doors or in some other part of the institution, or—during business hours on weekdays—at some therapy session.

In order to understand the daily life of the patients somewhat better, it is useful to know what the daily round of the rehab unit is like and what some typical patterns of patient activity are.

Most patients wake up (or are awakened) about 6:00 A.M. to start the process of getting ready for breakfast, which is served two hours later. This early hour enables the night nursing shift to take part in the morning preparation before the day shift comes on duty at 7:30. Some patients wash and take care of their personal needs in bed or in the bedside cubicle and others go to the bathroom.

A few patients sleep until a later time, and some until breakfast. Late sleepers include patients who are able to take care of their own personal needs and choose to let the washing-up go until the last minute, and those who need almost complete nursing care. It is the duty of the day shift to attend to the morning toileting and washing needs of the latter group, which is done after breakfast.

Those who get up early must occupy their time before 8:00 A.M. breakfast. A few go to Mass, while others sit in the corridors. For many, part of the time is occupied by arriving at the dining tables a long time before breakfast is served. By 7:30 many of them are already in place even though they have another half hour or longer to wait for their food.

Shortly after breakfast has been served, some of the patients who finish their meal early begin to disperse and move into the day room. Some eat quickly so as to beat the crowd to the bathroom. The therapeutic activities and organized diversional activities officially begin at 8:30, but very few patients go to these activities before 9:00. Often the ward routines make it impossible for them to go earlier, as the therapists often told us when we wondered why their therapy areas had few or no patients before 9:00. In any case, formal therapy programs take up only a small part of the morning for most patients and no time at all for others. Some of the patients may be examined by physicians on rounds, or have an interview with the social worker, but these are only occasional activities. The helpless patients are not bathed, dressed, and out of bed until midmorning.

The patients who eat in the dining area (and this is the great majority of them) gather at their tables for lunch between 11:30 and 12:00, a few of them coming in there even before 11:30. They eat their lunch between 12:00 and 12:30 and then disperse.

At 1:00 P.M. some go to therapy or other organized activities which last until about 4:00 (3:00 in the summer). They are not likely to be seen by physicians in the afternoon except for occasional special purposes. There are few routine nursing tasks during this time because almost all these routines are taken care of in the morning. Therefore the patients are even more on their own in the afternoon than in the morning. After

4:00 they are entirely on their own except for occasional programs put on by professional group workers or volunteers. Dinner is served at around 5:00 and the patients begin collecting again about a half hour earlier.

The most physically dependent patients are put to bed before the day shift leaves in mid-afternoon; others who are unable to get into bed by themselves are put to bed by a special crew around 7:00 or 8:00 P.M. Patients able to get into bed by themselves go to bed at various times, with a few late TV watchers still in the day room at 10:00 P.M.

There is no therapy and little organized activity on the rehab unit after dinner. Group work at one time had a regular Thursday evening program, and group work and occupational therapy together had a monthly cultural evening program. There are other occasional activities (usually some special hobbies) run by volunteers. There are also a few regular hospital-wide events which some patients attend—bingo in the recreation room, movies in the auditorium. However, most evenings patients are entirely on their own. On weekends, too, their time is their own except for the time consumed by nursing care routines and the occasional medical emergencies.

Patient groupings

TERRITORIES

Most rehab patients spend all or almost all their waking hours when not in therapy on the rehab unit and adjacent corridors. Observation reveals a number of subgroups in terms of location and activity.*

* We did not follow any one patient throughout the day, but made our observations of the entire hospital or of particular units within the hospital over a period of time and kept a record of the time and the activities of the patients observed as well as the interaction between patients (who talks to whom). Therefore, on a given patient we have a record of his activity and interaction for different times of the day

Some patients spend a large part of their waking hours in the day room. They may sit there for long periods doing nothing (or nothing which an observer can detect). Some use the day room in part as a place to meet their acquaintances. One group of women with a rather constant membership spent a substantial period of the day sitting in a semicircle in one corner in front of the television set. (We cannot say how much of the time they were actually watching TV. We noted that sometimes they had their eyes shut.)

Some patients spend much of their day in their ward cubicle. One or two of these are confined to bed. Most patients get away from their cubicles at least part of the day. The more time a patient spends in his cubicle, the more isolated he is from contact, both with his fellow patients and with the staff. His opportunity for catching physicians and social workers "on the run" is greatly reduced.

A few patients spend a relatively large amount of time parked in a wheelchair in the corridors outside the rehab unit. They see more of the staff and patients who come by than those who remain on the ward and thus may have the advantage of getting information or attention which they otherwise might not receive.

A minority of patients spend many of their waking hours off the rehab unit. About one-fourth of these usually—in some cases, always—are by themselves while they are off the ward. Their movement seems to be at least in part an escape from the round of life on the ward. These we call the "off-ward isolates."

In contrast, about three-fourths of this group go off the ward to join with other patients in the recreation room, to play cards

on different days beginning with the time patients get up in the morning to the time when the late TV watchers go to bed at night. By combining a series of such observations we constructed a "typical day," which does not represent any specific day of observation, but does represent a distribution of the patient's time and activities. We also constructed a "sociogram" of patient interaction patterns. See Appendix A for more details on procedure.

or eat in the canteen, or to sit around with other patients—often from other wards—and have a bull session. These conversation groups often fall into an obvious social category (e.g., age group, ethnic group). Thus, such off-ward congregating is an opportunity to find more of one's "own kind" than are available on the rehab unit itself. A few of these off-ward activists also participate in more formal hospital-wide activities—patients' committees and councils, patient newspaper, part-time jobs (usually at little or no pay).

INTERACTION GROUPS

The new patient coming on rehab does not find himself among an amorphous collection of fellow patients. Instead, he finds that, with the exception of those too ill to care about the company of others or those who are isolated by choice or by disability, patients on the ward belong to recognizable groups with definite reputations among the staff and other patients.

Of the 140 patients on whom we have sufficient information, we classified 60 as central members of interactional groups of three or more. Another 13 patients are classified as peripheral members of these same groups. Of the "leftovers," we classified 8 as isolates (virtually no observable interaction with their fellows) and 13 as near-isolates (few items of evidence of interaction). The remainder, about one-third of the total, are patients who cannot be called isolates but who do not fit clearly into any of the regularly interacting groups, although some of these patients (we definitely identified 6) spend a great deal of time in the company of patients from other parts of the hospital.

The largest of these interactional groupings are the "young adults" (a label used by staff and patients alike), who include all the male patients in their late teens and twenties, as well as several young women and older men among their peripheral membership. Even the severely disabled young men are included in the activities of this group in contrast to the situation among older patients where (as we shall see) the severely disabled are usually isolated. The young adults are the most clear-cut case we have of a single attribute (i.e., age grade) serving to organize a relatively stable social group and setting it off from the rest of the patient society. When the young adults go off the ward (as they frequently do), they interact chiefly with other young patients from other parts of the hospital. (However, a large proportion of the patients under thirty are concentrated on the rehab units.)

Other interactional groups organized around a single attribute are the small Italian and Spanish groups, who converse in their native tongue, but the organization of these groups is much looser—that is, they are more likely to interact with others outside of their group. The Italian group contains several severely deteriorated patients who never leave the ward. The Spanish group members often go off the ward to seek compatriots elsewhere.

One group consists entirely of Jewish patients, who might seem to be organized around their religion. Our observations suggest, however, that their ties are based largely on common recreational interests (although they are of course aware of their common ethnic affiliation), and a number of Jewish patients on rehab are not part of the group at all. Much of the Jewish group's recreation takes place in the hospital's recreation department or out-of-doors rather than on the ward.

The largest group next to the young adults are eight white women of middle-class background whom we have labeled the "respectable women." They are often among the leading participants in ward programs and are relatively well thought of by the staff. They go off the rehab unit much less often than the Jewish or young adult groups.

Three other groups are made up of lower-class Negro women (with the exception of a lone white woman), who spend almost all their time on the ward. The "old timers" (our label) are distinguished by their long careers on rehab, which sets them off from those who (relatively speaking) come and go. The "domestics" (our label) are a passive, conforming group with a background of servant-type work. The "alcoholics" (so labeled by the nursing staff) frequently hang around the day-room TV set conversing little with one another and still less with other patients. We never observed any of them drunk, but their reputation sticks to them. (Once again, we call the reader's attention to the fact that these groups are based on the relative amounts of interaction with one another, not on common attributes.)

The reader wishing more details on these groups, as well as several "splinter groups" not mentioned here, should consult Appendix C.

THE STARS

When our observations were plotted as a sociogram, four patients stood out as "stars." Only one was clearly a member of one of the interaction groups—Jane Bader of the respectable women. The remaining three have interaction patterns which are so scattered that they cannot be clearly identified with any single group.

Tom Ormsby and Gloria Crane were both active in group-work programs. In addition, Crane was an adviser to other patients, Ormsby a reformer and promoter. (These roles do not always go over well with other patients.) Crane, a Negro in her sixties, is in a white-collar occupation and has a very active social life outside the hospital. She had close connections with some members of the respectable women, Jewish, and domestic groups as well as with the other "stars" and many non-group members. Ormsby, a Negro in his forties, with an odd-job, "bum" background turned reformer, had close connections with the members of the respectable women, young adults, and old timers groups as well as with Crane and with other non-group members.

Sheila Rivera is more of an underground leader. A Puerto Rican in her mid-fifties, she had good relationships with many patients and lower-echelon staff throughout the hospital. She knew how to circumvent undesirable staff actions by subterfuge and direct pressure (more about this later). Rivera had close connections with the young adults, old timers, respectable women, and with several splinter groups, as well as with Crane and other non-group members and many patients and staff off the rehab unit.

The non-group position may perhaps serve to make these leaders more effective communicators and better able to move readily from one person and activity to another because they do not have to feel any obligation to first deliver their news and ideas or suggestions for activities to a few favored acquaintances before moving out to the larger patient society. Thus, it is quite possible that their lack of a solid group identification lends to their central position in the patient society on the rehab unit, although this is admittedly highly speculative.

THE ISOLATE END OF THE RANGE

We have classified eight of our total group of patients as isolates and another thirteen as near-isolates.

Eight of these patients are aphasics (five of them among the total isolates). These include all of the patients suffering from total or almost total aphasia who were on the ward during our period of observation except one man who was a member of the X group (described in Appendix C) and one woman who had a slight part in the domestic group after making some recovery from her aphasia. Another five of these people were regarded as mentally deteriorated or having very bizarre behavior. Since three of these are complete isolates, the eight complete isolates fall into the aphasic and bizarre deteriorated categories. Among the remaining nine, we have one patient who is blind, two who are completely bedridden, one who sleeps a large part of the day, and five who are extremely with-drawn for unknown reasons.

SEX AND ACTIVITY PATTERNS

Women dominate the informal interaction on the rehab ward. Although the women total only slightly higher than the men among those whom we observed and classified—seventy-two to sixty-eight—they make up the bulk of the informal groups on the unit. All the respectable women, old timers, domestics, the alcoholics, and the "newcomers" are women. Among the major groups the men are definitely ahead only in the young adult group, which is completely male in its central member-ship. Among the twenty-two isolates and near-isolates, nine-teen are men and only three are women.

On the other hand, if we divide the same 140 patients into ward and off-ward categories, it would seem at first sight that the men are more active:

	Male	Female
Rehab life circumscribed by ward unit	31	50
Substantial off-rehab life	26	11
Not clearly in either category	11	11

However, the great majority of the young adults on the unit are male. Also, one should not equate mobility with social activity. Seven out of the ten off-ward isolates are male, nine-teen out of the twenty-seven off-ward activists are male—about the same proportion in each case. Three out of the four ward leaders are women. Women predominate (sixteen out of twenty) in using the day room as a hangout (not counting the TV watchers who are *all* women), whereas the men pre-dominate (twelve out of twenty) in using the cubicle as a hangout. Thus, although men and women each dominate in given activities and territories, we cannot say in an over-all way that one sex is more active than the other on the rehab unit.

The patient class system

The reader has no doubt already remarked that the inter-action groups have reputations, which makes it possible to rank them in a rough way on a prestige scale.

A patient's prestige, as the notion is used here, consists largely of two elements—what he brings with him from the outside and what he achieves in terms of his activities in the hospital. Patients vary in their previous social reputation, some of them having a background of a stable family life, middle-class occupation, a home of their own, and similar respectability symbols, while at the other extreme some have reputations for alcoholism and for being transient "bums." Within the hospital the patient who takes a very active part in the informal activities of the patients' and/or staff-sponsored activities can enhance his reputation. Occasionally, a patient like Tom Ormsby enters with a social reputation as a "bum" and greatly improves his reputation among the staff and among the more "respectable" patients by espousing an active rehab philosophy and taking part in all patient activities. On the other hand, a patient with a high-level reputation on the outside may suffer a relatively poor reputation in the hospital because his disability prevents him from being a participant in the patient activities or renders him incontinent or irrational. Thus, brain damage or physical dependence not only makes one less desirable as a rehab candidate and makes it difficult to obtain care from the custodial staff (as we shall see in Chapter 4), but these factors may also damage one's standing with one's fellow sufferers and cause one to end up on much the same reputational stratum as someone who has been regarded as an uneducated lower-class unemployable throughout his adult life.

Using the reputational scheme suggested in the previous paragraph, the informal patient groups found on the rehab unit can be rated in a kind of class system. Indeed, they *are* so rated by many staff and patients, although of course they do not speak of it as a class system. In the "upper crust" we have the three non-group leaders, the respectable women, and the Jewish group. The alcoholics and many of the isolates make up the lower end of the scale. In between these two ends, we have the old timers, the domestics, the splinter groups, and the bulk of the non-group members (although a few of these would be rated quite high, especially by some of the staff). The newcomers are difficult to rate because they were not around long enough during our period of observation to make a definite place for themselves. The young adults are also difficult to rate under this scheme. They had a rather wide range in terms of social background and some important variations in their activity on the ward, the differences being largely a result of variation in the severity of their disabilities. However, on the rehab unit youth alone tends to rate high regardless of level of activity or social background, so any young people are bound to have an important place in the rehab program in the eyes of the staff and many of their fellow patients.

REPUTATION AND DRESS

An objective reputational indicator is the kind of clothing worn by the patients. Pajamas are usually hospital issue, although a few provide their own pajamas (or more correctly, they are provided by family members). They may also wear shirt and pants (in the case of the men) or dresses (in the case of the women) issued by the hospital and carrying an identification stamp showing that the clothing belongs to the hospital. Such hospital-issue clothing is likely to be a poorer fit than the clothing that the patient would obtain for himself and comes in a few standard patterns and colors. This makes a greater difference in the case of women than of men. Often it is difficult to distinguish the men wearing hospital clothes from those wearing their own clothes because they look very much alike. The women wearing hospital issue, however, stand out sharply from those wearing their own clothing since the dresses issued by the hospital seem to be more ill-fitting in comparison to the women's own clothes than the hospital issue given to men are in comparison to the clothing that the men would ordinarily wear.

Patients are frequently encouraged by occupational therapists, social workers, and some nurses to wear street clothes when they are out of bed rather than pajamas and robes, and if possible to wear their own clothing, which fits better and is less uniform in appearance than hospital issue. In fact, for a patient to wear his clothing is regarded by some staff members as an indicator of progress in rehabilitation. Considerable emphasis is put on clothing for participation in some formal activities.

The kind of clothing a patient wears closely matches other indications of reputational status. All of the central members of the respectable women and the Jewish groups as well as three out of four peripheral members of the Jewish group wear their own clothing rather than hospital issue. All of the central and peripheral members of the young adult group wear their own clothing except when some of the young adults who have to travel on a stretcher stay in their pajamas for part of the day. All of the central members of the old timers group commonly wear their own clothes, especially when they are in their wheelchairs.

On the other hand, six of the eight central and peripheral members of the domestic group and all in the alcoholic group commonly wear hospital issue. Among the splinter groups, all of the Spanish group wear their own clothing, but the great majority of the members of the other splinter groups wear hospital clothing. Among eighteen isolates and near-isolates on whom we have definite information, thirteen commonly wear hospital issue and only five wear their own clothing.

The newcomers group is split into two subgroups, one of which was around for a month or two when the second group came. It is interesting that three out of the four of the earlier group wear their own clothing and three out of the four of the latter group wear hospital issue, usually the hospital bedclothes. It is quite possible that this is a stage which many patients go through, and the fact that some of this group are already regularly wearing their own clothing may be an indicator that they will soon establish themselves as one of the higher reputational groups (or perhaps move into close association with already established groups).

REPUTATION AND STAFF-SPONSORED ACTIVITIES

An indicator of the articulation of the patient class system and staff values is provided by participation in staff-sponsored activities.

The rehab staff-sponsored activities on which we collected attendance records during our period of observation are the following:

Patient Planning Committee: Plan weekly entertainment and educational programs for patients. Attendance recorded for most of a year.

Rehab Newspaper: Written and printed by patients at widely spaced, irregular intervals. List of patients recorded for one issue only.

Cultural Evening: A monthly program of "cultural" events; this year dealing with talks and movies about foreign lands. Attendance recorded for a nine-month season.

Diversional Occupational Therapy: Projects in OT diversional shop—e.g., weaving, leather-work. Recorded regular users for three-month period.

Picnics: Outdoor food-and-game fests. Attendance recorded for all five picnics held in one summer.

Singing Group: Singing popular songs to accompaniment of a piano. Conducted by a Negro woman (volunteer) who worked as a messenger during the day. Attendance recorded at one session.

Women's Club: Attempt to stimulate any kind of activity on part of female patients who commonly hung around the ward—e.g., holding little parties, singing songs, pursuing hobbies. Attendance recorded at two sessions.

The chart to follow shows the number of participants in each of these activities according to the patient interaction category.

The activities are arranged from left to right on a staff-valued prestige scale. Members of the patient planning committee and the newspaper staff are both carefully selected by the group workers from what they regard as the more intelligent and responsible patients (although they sometimes "take a chance" on poorer risks as a form of social therapy). Participants in the cultural evening programs are also invited (in this case by group work and occupational therapy staff), but a deliberate effort is made to include a broader spectrum of patients, including some "borderline" cases, so that they might be given an incentive to practice grooming and dressing and participate in preparing exhibits, food, and invitations. Diversional OT is usually initiated at the patients' request, though some are encouraged by OTs or physicians to pursue this activity. Picnics are by invitation, but an effort was made over one summer to invite all who were deemed physically able to get about on foot or wheelchair without much help. Some did not attend when invited. The singing group is open to all. The women's group is chiefly aimed at the inactive females

PARTICIPATION BY INTERACTION GROUP MEMBERS IN STAFF-SPONSORED ACTIVITIES

	Patient Planning Committee[b]	Newspaper[c]	Cultural Evening[a]	Diversional OT	Picnics	Singing Group	Women's Club
Non-group leaders	3	1	2	—	3	—	—
Respectable women	4	—	4	2	3	2	3
Jewish	3	2	5	2	4	—	1
"Staff stars"[a]	—	—	3	—	—	—	—
Young adults	2	—	2	2	11	—	—
Old timers	—	—	—	—	1	—	—
Spanish	—	—	1	—	2	—	—
X group	—	1	1	—	1	—	1
Newcomers	—	—	—	—	—	—	6
Italian	—	—	—	1	2	—	—
Oriented off-rehab	1	1	—	—	—	—	—

"Other non-group"	—	2	3	3	5	3
Domestic	1	—	1	1	4	5
Alcoholic	1	—	1	1	—	5
Near-isolates	—	—	6	1	3	—
Isolates	—	—	—	—	1	—
Insufficient information	—	—	11	4	1	—

[a] Patients who were not leaders in the patient society, but who were very helpful to the group-work staff in running their program and thus tended to participate in group-work activities.

[b] All of the regular attenders at meetings of the Patient Planning Committee come from the Non-group leaders, Respectable women, Jewish, and Young adult groups.

[c] The more permanent members of the newspaper staff were all members of the Non-group leaders, Jewish, and X groups.

[d] Only six patients attended six or more cultural evening programs. Of these, two were members of the Jewish group, four were "Staff stars," and one was a domestic group member.

who hang out in the day room and in their cubicles. Some of its membership is the product of virtually forcible dragooning of the more disabled patients.

The patient categories are listed roughly from high to low prestige from top to bottom. Above the young adults are the clearly high-prestige categories; below the newcomers the clearly low-prestige categories. Between are the middle-range groups, which are difficult to order in a hierarchy.

Note that top participants weigh more heavily at the left of the chart; bottom participants more heavily at the right. Even the effort to include the more neglected patients in cultural evenings left out the domestics, alcoholics, and extreme isolates, precisely the ones who most often wear hospital clothing and tend to be carelessly dressed and groomed. Though a wider range of patients becomes involved in the lower-rated activities, refusals to attend the picnics are heavy among the alcoholics and isolates, and the women's club gets its heavy representation among lower-status patients only because many are pushed, protesting, to the day room at the appointed time.

The selection, both by staff and by the patients themselves, tends to keep patients from lower-status categories out of higher-status activities, and works in many cases to keep the lowly from any formal activity—certainly no surprise to anyone familiar with the effects of stratification in our larger society.

Disability and the limitation of activity

The brief description of the isolates and near-isolates earlier in this chapter showed that these patients are for the most part severely disabled. The same physical, psychological, and social disabilities which often cut patients off from relationships with their fellows also limit their activity and reduce their ability to bargain with the staff for assistance in maintaining an active life.

Of the eighty-one patients whose lives are circumscribed by

the ward unit, nineteen are unable to get around by themselves in a wheelchair or by any other method, or have such a
limited ability to move themselves about that in practice they
cannot go far in any direction. The importance of this factor
is underlined in the sharp change that took place in several of
the activity patterns. Lloyd Priest was seen much less often
hanging out in the day room and Sara Kent was found much
less often in her cubicle once they had received their electric
wheelchairs. John Green and Giuseppe Bozzo are both cate-
gorized here in the hospital-wide activities group, but there
were periods of time when these two men were suffering from
severe decubitis ulcers (open skin lesions) and during these
periods they were much more likely to be found on the ward,
especially in their cubicles, despite the fact that they had both
been provided with stretchers which they could wheel around.
The greater difficulty in moving around with a stretcher is
sufficient to significantly reduce off-ward traveling.

We classified another fourteen of these eighty-one as
"limited sociability" along with five of the seven who hang
out in the corridor outside the rehab unit and five of the ten
who have relatively isolated off-rehab patterns. The following
is a table of the non-socializing characteristics of these twenty-
four patients (some of them could be put in more than one
of these categories):

Categories

Severe difficulty in oral communication	12
(usually aphasia resulting from a stroke)	
Considered crazy or mentally retarded by others	5
Extreme psychological withdrawal	5
Sharp ethnic isolation	2

Physical helplessness and the various limitations on sociability, therefore, account for close to half of those people who
spend most of their time around the ward or go off the rehab

unit mainly to escape from interaction with others on the ward. The very dependent patients and those of limited sociability are dependent on others to initiate sociable interaction with them. Their isolation is physical and sociological, not simply a matter of personality make-up. The operating structure of the hospital and the unit contribute to imposing isolation upon them.

Another way of putting this is to say that relative isolation and restricted activity are not always a matter of choice. True, several of those who sit in their cubicles most of the day want a great deal more privacy than the hospital situation affords and hide out in their cubicle with curtain drawn as the best possible solution. However, others are there because they cannot move by themselves and cannot find ward staff who are willing and able to move them to another location at the time they wish. Some of those who spend most of their day in the day room can sit up in a wheelchair, but are unable to move about. They are helped out of bed in the morning, wheeled to the day room by a nurse or aide and left there for a large part of the day. To provide some daily variety in their location and association with others, such people would have to call upon the ward staff repeatedly during the day to be moved. Such frequent requests (say, as much as once an hour) quickly bring a reprimand from nurses and aides who regard this kind of catering to a patient's "whims" as beyond the reasonable call of duty. Take, for example, Mrs. Bauer's (head nurse) statement on a demanding patient (from our field notes on a staff meeting):

> Mrs. Bauer entered the discussion and gave Black (a psychologist) an instance of why she thought a psychological evaluation was necessary (for Mrs. Salmanoff, a patient). It turns out that last Saturday morning the patient was in the day room watching television. Bauer came into the room and the patient beckoned to her, and Bauer went over to see what she wanted. The patient wanted her to either turn off the TV or move her chair farther away from it. Bauer did not want

to turn the TV off since other patients were watching it. She therefore moved the chair four feet away, over by a post which she described as "a good position." At that time another patient called to Bauer and she went over to attend to the other patient's needs. Salmanoff called Bauer back and wanted to be moved two feet farther down toward the ward. Bauer told her that she could not do this because if she moved her there, she would be blocking the passageway. The patient then asked to be moved back closer to the TV. Within five minutes, therefore, Salmanoff had asked to be moved three times. Bauer says it is because of this kind of behavior that the aides won't go near this patient.

The aphasic or the extremely withdrawn patient, of course, cannot even make such requests infrequently and is likely to be left to himself except when specific medical procedures or routine ward procedures are carried out.

That relative isolation and inactivity do not necessarily go with extreme handicap is shown by the experience of two of the patients. Both are men with so little muscle strength that they can scarcely move their wheelchairs and such weak voices that they can be understood only if one is close by and the noise level is low. One—a teen-aged boy—was adopted by the young adults. They often pushed him to other parts of the hospital to join their group. They made him part of their conversations and frequently played cards with him. The other— a man in his thirties—was adopted by an older man who is ambulatory and physically strong (for this population). This "big brother" spent a large part of each day with him, pushed him around the hospital in his wheelchair, took him to organized activities and helped him to participate (e.g., held bingo cards). During our period of systematic observation of activities, both these men were rated with the "activists." Without the help of their fellow patients they would certainly have been among the isolated and inactive group.

Most of the more severely disabled patients are not adopted by their fellow patients as were these two men. Except for occasional minor favors, they are left alone by other patients who are having trouble enough salvaging their own shattered lives. The ward staff's definition of their appropriate tasks does not include hour-to-hour personal service to patients. For one of the patients (or one of the professional or administrative staff members) to expect such service is seen as an unwarranted imposition on their workday. Therefore, requests by patients to the ward staff to be moved or to be helped in some other way to change their activity (e.g., turning on the radio or changing the station) are discouraged by the staff, and service is frequently refused or ignored when a request *is* made. Only on occasions when family members or friends visit (which for many patients is never) or volunteers help out with a formal program (e.g., taking patients in wheelchairs and stretchers to the movie theater) can the severely disabled patient expect relief from this pattern of inactivity.

Insofar as we look upon Farewell Hospital (including the rehab unit) as the patient's home rather than simply a place for specialized therapy, an important part of patient care (important, that is, to the patient) is being left out. The physical and psychological handicaps of some of the patients severely restrict the activities they can engage in on their own. The work definitions of the ward staff exclude much of what is vitally important to the disabled patient. Such a patient finds himself in a situation where some of his most important needs are nobody's business.

Patients and   4
their caretakers

Let us take a closer look at the caretakers who are so often condemned by both patients and professional workers. How do they fit into the hospital and rehab scheme? Just how important are they compared to other staff?

One way of answering the last question is to imagine the effects of a work stoppage among different groups of staff. Let us first imagine a work stoppage among all the physical therapists, occupational therapists, speech and hearing therapists, and social workers. What would happen? If these staff groups went on strike late Friday afternoon or before a holiday, nothing would happen right away. In fact, the patients would not even notice that anything unusual had occurred. The next workday, some patients on active therapy programs would be annoyed to find that the PT gymnasiums and OT shops were closed and would complain about their progress being delayed. Other patients would breathe a sigh of relief because they were going to be allowed to rest rather than being put through an exercise program which they really didn't want. A few patients in the midst of negotiating their discharge from the hospital would be upset because the social worker who is handling the paper work is not available. But they would be no worse off than the patients whose social worker goes off on a month's vacation without telling them in advance, leaving them sitting around waiting for their discharge until she returns. If the strike lasted several weeks, let us say, one or two discharges might be held up and therapy for several dozen patients would be delayed, though some patients already well into their therapy programs would be able to carry on by themselves if somebody would unlock the doors to the therapy rooms and put out the equipment.

Now let us imagine a work stoppage on the part of the aides and the ward nurses. Everyone concerned would recognize this as a crisis requiring immediate action. The more helpless patients would soil their beds. No food would be served. Those unable to get out of bed without help would not even have water unless their more able fellows brought it to them. The therapy program would be reduced because the more severely disabled patients would never arrive at the therapy areas. Dressings would not be changed and no medications given. Some corrective action would have to be taken within hours, even if the work stoppage began on a weekend or at night. Supervisory personnel and volunteers would be rushed in to take care of the most urgent ward tasks and they would have to continue to cover the wards until the regular ward workers returned.

Despite their obvious necessity for the operation of the institution and the urgency of their tasks, the ward personnel find themselves at the bottom of the rehab status heap, often despised by the professional specialists.

The caretakers and the team

The caretakers are quite sharply set off from the professional rehab staff. Few have professional training. The unit supervisor and usually the daytime charge nurses on the male and female wards are registered nurses. Sometimes the nurse in charge of the whole unit in the evening is an RN. There will be several practical nurses on the day shift and one on the evening and night shifts if there is no RN on duty. The great majority of the ward workers are aides. They carry out their daily routines with little financial reward or acknowledgment of their effort from the institution they work for, the patients they take care of, or the professional staff they work with, which looks down on them from a distance. They are assigned dining facilities separate from the professional and administrative employees and wear uniforms which set them off from other workers. They never participate in team meetings or any other decision-making groups on rehab. Even the professional nurses who do usually attend the team meetings participate less than the representatives of any other specialty. They give only a very brief formal report when their turn comes—a report which often represents a minute and uninteresting part of the information they actually have about the patient—and sit silently through the many lively discussions and arguments which engage the rest of the team. Only when the work of the ward staff is directly attacked by one of the team members do they enter the discussion in an effort to defend themselves, their colleagues, and their subordinates. Their opinions on how to treat the patients are seldom asked for and their interpretations of patient behavior are seldom taken seriously by the psychologists, social workers, and therapists.

The chasm between the professional rehab staff and the caretaker staff is intensified by the fact that the professionals frequently criticize the ward staff for not doing their job right. Sometimes this criticism is directed at specific mistakes. A paraplegic developed skin ulcers because the nursing personnel did not turn him often enough or did not properly massage the pressure areas; a patient's wound became infected because they did not change his dressing; a patient is really not incontinent as labeled by the nurses, but simply is not being taken to the toilet when he should be; a patient is not developing the skills in dressing himself which he learned in OT because the aides pull his pants on for him instead of standing by while he attempts it himself; a patient is not showing up for scheduled PT because the aides are taking too long to get him ready in the morning; a patient is not able to attend the evening group-work program because the nurses insist on putting him to bed at 7:00 P.M.—and so on.

Sometimes the criticism becomes much more sweeping. Nurses are too authoritarian; they are too concerned with petty routines rather than the important needs of the patients; they maintain rigid ward schedules which interfere with other parts of the rehab program; they are lazy and do not want to do their work. Therapists sometimes talk as if their efforts to retrain patients were being deliberately sabotaged by the ward staff.

The nursing staff is well aware that they are the butt of general criticism. They are not only forced to be defensive about their part in the program, but are suspicious of any overtures toward cooperative ventures. The sporadic efforts of PT, OT and group work to launch "ward programs" are received unenthusiastically by the ward staff. When professional staff members venture from their offices and therapy rooms to the ward to give suggestions and instructions on how to care for the patients, the nursing personnel often view this as "interference." ("I don't tell them how to give exercises and how to counsel patients; why should they tell me how to run a ward?")

Actually, the efforts of the professionals to actively intervene in ward operations are few and far between. They usually occur only when there is a medical or social crisis involving a patient, the news of which spreads outside the ward. Also, some specific consideration may be given to what is happening to a patient on the ward when it becomes obvious that there is an extreme discrepancy between his physical ability on the ward and his ability in the therapy sessions (e.g., he readily transfers from bed to wheelchair for the therapist, but tells the aides that he is incapable of doing so). The nursing supervisor may then be provided with suggestions which she may or may not be able to apply. The professionals rarely come on the ward to consult directly with the nurses and aides and to see concretely what the problems are. They exert even less control over the afternoon and night shifts whom they often accuse of undermining treatment efforts. They cannot understand why the daytime supervisor cannot assure them that a patient will be turned every two hours by the night shift. Yet none of the professional staff ever comes on the ward during the evening or night to see what is happening or to discuss the matter directly with the nursing personnel on those shifts.*

* In the same way, the P.M. and night shifts escape the influence of a new program in the mental hospital studied by Anselm Strauss, et al. The daytime nursing staff was won over to the "patient government" approach introduced by several psychiatrists, but the other two shifts continued their usual practices, often in direct contradiction to the principles which had been laid down by the daytime group for dealing with the patients. Here, too, the professional staff—despite their complaints about the P.M. and night ward workers—never bothered to come around after their regular hours. (Based on field notes from the study reported in part in Anselm Strauss, et al., *Psychiatric Ideologies and Institutions* (The Free Press, 1964).

The caretakers and their charges

Those who carry out the menial tasks of patient care are often
from a social background similar to that of the patients.
Nearly all are Negro, Puerto Rican, or European immigrants
of low social status. They sometimes form friendships with
patients of like origin or characteristics. In fact, several of the
old timers—middle-aged patients who had been on rehab for
several years—would never have lasted as long as they did on
this unit without the sympathetic support of the ward staff.
However, the potential number and depth of such friendships
are severely curtailed by factors which tend to create mutual
feelings of hostility between the caretakers and the patients.

To begin with, the patient often arrives on the ward ex-
pecting the same type of nursing service he had in a previous
hospital. The very fact that he is expected to attend to his own
needs insofar as possible frequently causes him to perceive the
aides as a lazy group who are not doing their duty by him.
If, in fact, the patient is dependent on the aides for help and
does not receive it, this image of the aide is reinforced. It is
significant that the most bitter criticism of the nursing staff
which is heard from patients comes from the severely disabled
who are dependent on others for many of their bodily needs
as well as their involvement in social activities. Those who are
mobile and able to care for their own needs tend to ignore the
nursing staff except when there is a disagreement about the
observance of ward rules. ("I don't bother them; they don't
bother me.") Those who cannot afford to ignore the ward
workers often accuse them of not doing their work and not
caring about the patients.

Because the aide is bound by hospital-wide schedules of
feeding, arousing patients in the morning and bedding them
down at night, she frequently has no control over the time
certain services can be rendered to a patient. In the creation of

hostile feelings, however, the services which the aide may not be able to give because of hospital regulations are less important than the unwanted services she frequently must perform in response to a telephone call requesting the removal of a patient from the ward. Communication channels are such that in fact it is the aide who often tells the patient about discharge and bodily removes him elsewhere. In like manner, it is the aide who frequently tells patients about appointments they must keep, interviews they must attend, and meetings or clinics at which their presence is desired. Since these announcements are usually news to the patient, who may have other plans or desires, the aide bears the brunt of patient displeasure as the visible agent who is forcing him to do something he does not understand or may have no interest in doing.

The visibility of the aides and nurses and the invisibility of other staff members place the aides and nurses in an especially vulnerable position to receive the main thrust of patient reactions to the institution. Other staff members can readily escape from the complaining patient, but the aide whose work is primarily on the ward itself has no office to retreat to and is more dependent on observable methods of handling patients' requests, needs, and gripes. She may be neither more nor less conscientious about pursuing her work than anyone else on the staff, but because her activities are more readily seen and felt by patients, complaints about her are more clearly articulated, and she becomes a ready scapegoat for the errors of omission and commission for which she herself may be responsible, as well as those of others for whom she is only the messenger of bad news (from the patient's point of view) or the hired hand who does the dirty work of patient care. Further, the services needed from the aide are often urgent and more acutely felt if not given immediately, whereas the services rendered by other disciplines are often less urgent and can be postponed with less distress to the patient. (Compare, for example, the need of a bedpan to the need of a prosthetic leg.)

Caretakers and activities of daily living

"Activities of daily living" (ADL) is a phrase commonly used in rehabilitation therapy. ADL are the activities we all engage in to take care of our bodily needs and to present ourselves to our fellows decently groomed and attired. These activities, which for most of us are a taken-for-granted routine, are a serious problem of management to the severely disabled person. If that person is a patient on a rehab unit, his difficulty with ADL is also a problem to the rehab staff.

In a sense, the improvement of a patient's ability to care for own needs is the central task of the entire rehab staff. The work of the PTs and the OTs is intended primarily to improve a patient's strength and coordination, increase his neuromuscular skills, and provide him with assistive devices to enable him to better perform his ADL. The social worker's efforts to place a patient outside the institution are heavily dependent on the patient's competence in caring for his needs. However, it is the ward worker's schedule that is most continuously and intimately affected by a patient's skill or lack of skill in performing his ADL.

To an occupational therapist, a patient's inability to feed himself is a professional problem to which she devotes her expertise during a regularly scheduled period during business hours of each non-holiday weekday. To the ward aide, the patient's inability to feed himself means that time must be taken at every meal to feed him. To the physical therapist, a patient's inability to transfer from wheelchair to toilet and back is again a professional problem to be worked on at scheduled sessions—over many months, if necessary. To the nurse or aide, the patient's handicap means that he must be helped to and from the toilet repeatedly each day, and that his bed or clothes and his person must be cleaned up if the ward workers delay too long in taking care of him.

Therapists have considerable control over their schedule. The beginning of therapy programs for new patients may be delayed if the therapist's schedule is full. On the ward, all patients must be cared for no matter whether there are ten helpless cases or twenty helpless cases at a given time, although nurses do exert some pressure to avoid having "too many" difficult patients at one time. External delays of months in placing a patient in the community is irritating to a social worker; to ward personnel it means providing care for the patient for months after his therapy is completed and he is simply awaiting discharge.

From their view, ward workers must get their routines done, avoid obvious disorder, and keep from being overwhelmed with work. In this framework, the patient is a potential source of disruption, added labor, and disturbance. He must be "managed" so that his demands do not get out of line and so that his behavior does not precipitate crises.

If the patient is new on the ward, he must be taught the customary behaviors and ordering of relationships which express the values of the ward staff. These translate the traditional emphasis of rehab on maximum independence in ADL in such a manner that the work of the custodial care of patients may be done and patients themselves may contribute to keeping the work load of the ward within reasonable limits as defined by the ward employees.* The education of the patient into the rehab philosophy and its demands upon the patient begins at the time he is wheeled onto the wards on a stretcher or wheelchair. The central focus of this education is on activities concerned with feeding, dressing, grooming, toileting, and moving from one position to another, and the educational techniques used may best be analyzed in terms of the ward organization for meeting these daily needs of patients.

* Cf. Rue Bucher and Leonard Schatzman, "The Logic of the State Mental Hospital," *Social Problems,* vol. 9 (Spring 1962), pp. 337–349.

SHELTER

The first need of a new patient is for a bed. A cubicle with a bed is assigned to the patient shortly after his arrival. On the female ward a cubicle adjacent to the nurses' station is reserved for all new patients and is officially referred to as the admitting bed. It serves as a temporary neutral zone where patients are placed until examined by a physician on duty and the nursing staff can evaluate the patient prior to a more permanent assignment. Usually patients remain here for only a day or two. A formal admitting bed is not found on the male ward. Males are immediately assigned a permanent cubicle. Placement in a cubicle also means placement on one of the three sections of the ward which radiate out from the nurses' station like three spokes from the hub of a wheel. Assignment to a section is primarily based on the patient's degree of cleanliness. In all sections the two beds closest to the nurses' station are reserved for the more dependent patients.

The most independent patients are assigned to the front section of the ward, which serves as a passageway to and from the day room for all patients and through which one must pass in order to reach the other two sections of the ward and the nurses' station. By common agreement among the nursing staff, this section is regarded as a showcase. Since the patients are relatively independent of the need for care, they are out of their cubicles early in the morning and for most of the day, which facilitates making and keeping this section presentable to the public eye for longer periods of time than is possible in sections with patients requiring considerable care.

The most dependent patients are assigned to one of the two remaining sections. The third section is allocated to patients who are in between the most dependent and independent groups. There is some tendency to place patients in this section who have problems in speech due to physical causes or deficiencies in English or who have a past history of alcoholism or psychological aberrations such as past suicide attempts, hallucinations, or temper tantrums. Although a given section may contain all kinds of patients, the general trends are as described. The data have been derived from personal observation on the ward, a careful census of patients on each section over a period of several weeks, and conversations with nursing personnel. The sharpest contrast is between the front section and the two back sections. The female ward is more clearly organized along these lines than is the male ward.

Intra-ward transfers are frequent. They are most frequent on the female ward not only because all the women are moved in and out of an admitting bed, but also because the organization of the ward is based on a system of moving women to the front section as they become increasingly independent. On both the male and the female wards the patient's appearance is a factor in transfer and can serve to move a messy or dirty patient to a back ward or to advance a neat patient to a front ward. In this manner the location of patients on the ward is one index of the nurses' evaluation of him as a person as well as an indication of his physical condition and the division of labor among the nursing personnel. Patients seem to be unaware of the implications of intra-ward transfer. They sometimes react negatively or positively to their new location, but when questioned as to the reason for a change, they state that they do not know. Since they are quite aware of the significance of transfer to various wards off the rehab service and speak quite frankly about it, it seems unlikely that they are trying to hide the meaning of intra-ward transfer from the researcher.

FEEDING

In addition to the location of his cubicle, the physical arrangements for feeding patients also allow a patient to make a series of transitions. Patients eat in a dining area located in the large day room and separated from the main portion of the day room by a three-foot-high partition. Males and females share the day room and the dining facilities. All patients who can feed themselves and are not on stretchers are assigned a place at the dining-room tables. Special diet tables are provided for diabetics and others whose diet is subject to control. A table for sloppy eaters is provided in the rear of the dining room until they gain sufficient physical control in feeding themselves so that they can be moved to another table. In addition to the above factors, the assignment of seats is intended to separate patients whom the nurses would prefer not to have associate with one another (e.g., alcoholics).

Patients unable to feed themselves are segregated from the dining area and eat in the main portion of the day room away from the other patients. They are fed by aides and may be completely or partially dependent on the aide and/or assistive devices. (Such assistive devices are dishes, eating utensils, slings, etc., which are especially made to enable a handicapped person to feed himself when he is unable to do so without these aids.) Although stretcher patients may be independent in feeding, they too are segregated from the main dining area because of the lack of space for stretchers at the tables and the fact that they need lower tables than are found in the dining area.

One can make progress within the dining area itself or from outside the area into it. It is also possible to make a third transition from eating in one's cubicle to eating in the day room. The only patients allowed to eat in their cubicles are patients who are sick, provided the nurses do not think they are malingering, or so incapacitated that they cannot be placed on a wheelchair or stretcher. Every effort is made to get these incapacitated patients out of bed as soon as possible. When they are able to come to the day room for meals, they begin by having lunch outside the dining area. They are invariably patients requiring assistance in eating.

Whether or not they will progress to three meals a day in the day room depends on sufficient improvement in their physical ability so that they require a minimum of assistance in getting out of or into bed. The responsibility for getting severely dependent patients into or out of bed falls on the nursing shift with the greatest number of nurses. Since this is the day shift, which comes on duty at 7:30 A.M. and leaves at 3:30 P.M., they cannot get these patients out of bed before serving breakfast or serve dinner to them before putting them to bed. The patients therefore are served these two meals in bed.

DRESSING, GROOMING, AND TOILET TRAINING

Dressing and grooming is a third ADL which permits transitions to occur based on physical independence. The careful bathing and dressing of patients who are to appear at staff meetings is but one indication of the value placed on the patient who appears clean and attractive. The potential relationship between a good appearance and assignment to a ward section has already been noted. Patients will be provided with assistive devices (e.g., elastic shoelaces, long-handled shoehorns) to enable them to dress themselves. As they issue hospital clothing to patients, nurses frequently use extra trinkets or more attractive items as a method of coaxing a patient into good grooming or rewarding him for progress already made. Dressing and grooming provide a dual means of ranking patients; those who are independent in dressing themselves are ranked more highly than those dependent in this respect; those who are neatly dressed are ranked higher than the carelessly or slovenly dressed. The ideal is the patient who can dress independently and has his own attractive clothes to wear.

Closely related to problems in grooming is the problem of incontinence. Incontinence is taboo on the ward and a serious offense when it occurs. Patients unable to control their bodily elimination are quickly told that "over here we don't put up with that" and are threatened with removal from the ward if they do not improve. Toilet training for such patients consists of scolding them, placing them on a regular schedule for going to the bathroom, and when necessary teaching them the art of transferring from a wheelchair to a toilet seat so as to eliminate the need for bedpans and help from the nurses' aides during the daytime. A desire to learn independence in toileting is reinforced by the fact that help is not available when a patient needs relief and he suffers discomfort until help comes or, if he is unable to hold out, a scolding for incontinence.

THE ROLE OF THE WHEELCHAIR

The emphasis of ward organization on physical mobility and transition is made possible by the fact that nearly all patients have a means of transportation—namely, the wheelchair. As soon as possible after their arrival, patients are expected to be up and out of their cubicles. The first step in this direction for the more severely disabled patient is to get him up in a wheelchair for a few hours each day and to wheel him into the day room for a meal or to watch television. For the majority of patients who do not need to be pushed around, instruction in the art of wheeling a wheelchair is provided by nurses' aides or other patients. Learning to wheel the chair competently is crucial for successful adaptation to ward life; for the majority of patients it provides the only means of getting around the hospital and off the wards without the nurses' aides, since only a very few patients can walk by themselves or on crutches.

Control of the work load

The ward workers' efforts to reduce the burden produced by patients' lack of ADL skills often fall into three categories:

1. Teach the patient the skills needed to care for himself.
2. Take care of the patient's needs for him.
3. If the patient is too great a burden, get rid of him by having him removed from the ward.

The third of these alternatives will be discussed in the next section. Let us now look at the first two, which operate as a dialectic of work control.

If the patient can be taught to transfer from bed to wheelchair and from wheelchair to toilet and back, the aides will no longer have to help him and their total work load will have been reduced by that degree. Also, the patient will have been rendered more independent—one of the major goals of the rehab program. However, teaching a patient the necessary skills for transfer may in itself take a great deal of time and, in some cases, is never successful. Therefore, the ward worker must decide in the case of a given patient whether it is worth pursuing.

If a patient cannot pull up his pants himself, the quickest way to get him dressed is to pull his pants up for him. But if you always do this, he will never learn to do it himself. How much time is it worth spending to stand by giving suggestions and occasional help while the patient laboriously strives to pull on his pants? Does it pay to put a great deal of time into training patients toward greater independence when, if you are very successful, they will be discharged from rehab and replaced by a more dependent patient who will increase the work load again?

The dilemma of whether to teach patients to do things for themselves or do things for them is influenced by the staffing and the kinds of patients on the ward at a given time. If the number of severely dependent patients increases sharply (as it did at one point on the female unit), nurses and aides who have been spending much of their time trying to teach ADL skills find that they cannot get through their daily routines unless they abandon much of the teaching. The same is true when the exigencies of scheduling leave a ward shorthanded.

The two different approaches to accomplishing the patients' ADL not only form a dialectic of counteracting forces among the ward workers, but pose potential and sometimes active conflict with professional therapists.

If a nurse or aide encourages a patient to try to transfer from wheelchair to toilet by himself, the physical therapist (if she hears about it) may contend that the patient is not ready for independent transfer, that the ward worker is risking a fall and serious injury to the patient. In such a case, the PT may maintain that it is her job to teach the patient to transfer and the ward workers should continue to help him until she (the PT) lets them know that the patient can safely transfer by himself.

On the other hand, for some tasks for which the patient is undergoing training, the therapist may want him to have an opportunity to practice on the ward. If an occupational therapist is trying to teach a patient to feed himself with special utensils she has devised, she may want him to begin eating some of his meals at least partly on his own. The aide who is pressed for time and does not want to wait while the patient very slowly works his way through his meal (and have to clean up his spilled food afterward) may prefer to feed him by spooning the food into his mouth.

Therapists sometimes try to deal with this dilemma by coming to the ward themselves to carry on part of the retraining in a more realistic life situation. The PTs have occasional programs in transfer and ambulation on the ward. OTs sometimes come at times when patients are dressing or eating to help them with these tasks. But such efforts are always short-lived. The therapists prefer their own work areas and when pressed for time and forced to make a choice, it is always the ward programs which are cut out.

Take, for example, the case of a patient with grossly weak-

ened muscles whom an OT was trying to retrain to feed himself with the help of some assistive devices. When the patient
complained that the aides never gave him a chance to eat by
himself, the OT came every lunch time to take over the task
of feeding him in accordance with her teaching program,
although she did not provide this service at breakfast or dinner
because these meals did not fall within her working hours.
After a few weeks, the OT went on vacation and no one else
took over her job. By the time she returned, other tasks had
piled up and she never got back to any mealtime training for
this patient. Thus, despite the exhortations of the OT, the
ward workers found that the bulk of her work had been
placed in their hands.

Who belongs on rehab?

Like caretakers in other types of institutions, the nursing personnel on rehab develop notions of the kind of patient rehab
is designed to serve and what may reasonably be expected of
those assigned to rehab as patients.*

Rehab is not for the care of the helpless. If a patient is helpless when he first comes on the ward but has the potential for
considerable improvement in the near future (e.g., a recent
"cerebral vascular accident"—CVA—or "stroke" victim), he
may be tolerated for a time. But long-term helplessness is seen
as inappropriate, and nurses will make an effort to have the
patient transferred to another unit. They particularly feel that
patients who are incontinent or who fall frequently, thereby
creating a great deal of work for them, are poor choices for
the rehab wards, and they sometimes request the removal of
such patients from rehab. They are unlikely to be successful in

* For a similar conception of staff images of given wards and the
patients appropriate to them, see Anselm Strauss, et al., *Psychiatric
Ideologies and Institutions,* pp. 278–288.

this effort if, by the time they realize that the patient's incontinence or falling is a chronic problem, he has already been established on a therapy program and the decision on discharge is largely in the hands of the therapists, social workers, and supervising physicians who often dismiss nurses' complaints as unimportant.

Patient behavior which the ward staff deems clearly undesirable and inappropriate to a rehab setting and which shows up at an early stage of the patient's stay on the unit will often shorten his stay. The following categories of behavior have this effect:

1. Overt mental disturbance or incompetence.

2. Aggressive nonconformity.

3. Refusal of patients to help themselves when they are physically able to.

Eleven of the sixty patients in our sample were regarded by the custodial staff as mentally unbalanced or mentally incompetent (the latter usually being brain-damaged CVAs). Eight out of twenty (in our sample of sixty) with the shortest stay on rehab fell in this group, with the remaining forty accounting for only three. Nine of the sixty patients were considered by the custodial staff as being aggressively noncomforming. Five of these were among the twenty with the shortest stay. Six of the sixty patients were regarded by the nursing staff as refusing to help themselves when they were physically able to do so. Four of these are part of the twenty with the shortest stay. Altogether, twelve of these twenty short-stay patients had at least one of these undesirable characteristics. Only nine out of the remaining forty had one of these characteristics.

During the early weeks of patients' stay on rehab, nursing personnel and medical residents have an important part in decisions concerning the patients' disposition, even though nursing plays a very small role in the formal team meetings. The patients are not well known to the therapy staffs simply because they have been there for such a short time. In our sample, seven patients never received any therapy at all; five did not even come up for the first team meeting. The therapy staff therefore was not familiar with them and had no effective hand in the decision about their disposal. These decisions were initiated by the nursing and medical resident staffs.

Physicians of higher authority have to approve all transfers or discharges, but if the nurses or ward doctors give relevant arguments why patients should not be there, the supervising physician is likely to accept this argument if there is no contradictory evidence. If the patient behaves in a way that makes him difficult to manage, such a recommendation is more likely to get him removed from the ward quickly. When a physician speaks of a "problem patient," he means that the patient is a problem in ward management and he received details about such problems from the ward nursing staff who must deal with the patients throughout the day, day after day. The patient who is grossly insubordinate, abusive, refuses to try to help with his own care, or who presents an extremely difficult problem in nursing care right at the very beginning is not likely to last long on rehab.

Behavioral aberrations in such patients may be used as a basis for moving them to the psychiatric wards, while bizarre behavior on the part of the patients who give no other trouble may be tolerated for many months. Symptoms of physical pathology may also be used as grounds for very quickly moving such patients off to a medical unit with no recommendation that they return to rehab at a later time; similar symptoms in a longer-stay patient in whom the rehab staff has already made some investment is more likely to be tolerated while an attempt is made to treat his disorder on the rehab unit, or, if he is transferred to another ward for special treatment, he is taken back on rehab after the other treatment has been completed. The psychiatrist, too, relies very heavily on nursing and ward doctor reports in the patients' charts for making recommendations about the placement of patients and thus the custodial staff can influence the psychiatrist's decision in those cases where the psychiatrist is consulted.

In the early days of a patient's stay on the rehab wards, the consequences of an arrangement which leaves both the patient and the ward staff out of the decision-making process with respect to patient selection and care are particularly apparent. During his first few days on rehab, the patient's fate is largely in the hands of the ward staff who have the responsibility of taking care of him. Misunderstanding of the patient's genuine need for help on the part of the ward employees and the patient's own lack of knowledge of what the ward staff expects can and often does result in acrimonious relations between the two groups.

Usually lacking in outside agents from among his family and friends, and often unable to act on his own behalf, the rehab patient at Farewell is in an especially powerless position to contribute to the enhancement of his position and the service which he can reasonably expect to receive from the ward staff. The patient who is physically independent can partially overcome this lack of power by attending to his own needs and avoiding demands upon the ward staff as much as possible. The highly dependent patient, however, is severely handicapped in caring for himself and must often make persistent demands to obtain even minimal services.

Whether he is dependent or independent, the patient must not grossly violate the ward staff's image of the good patient by becoming a "trouble-maker" who for physical or other reasons causes undue work for the nursing staff or threatens their authority. Those who do become "trouble-makers" for any one of a variety of reasons are likely to be removed from the ward and the rehab program, sometimes before they have been evaluated by the professional rehab team.

For the patient who believes rehab to be his best possibility for leaving Farewell or making life there more tolerable, such a removal may be viewed as a disaster. Even those patients who are unaware of the potential contribution of rehab to their welfare may suffer ill effects from a premature or arbitrary dismissal from the rehab program. Those who survive the first month or longer and become established on a therapy program can be less concerned with the opinion of the caretakers provided the therapeutic staff is satisfied with their progress. For these patients, rehab becomes something more than a routine life on the wards and involves at least a limited contact with the therapeutic life offered by the rehab team.

The team 5

The "team" which holds out hope of return to physical "normality" to those who survive the ward initiation is primarily a medical team dominated by medical practices, organization, and authority. The physicians decide which patients should be selected for rehab, what types of therapy they should be given, and when they have reached the point where they may be discharged from the program. True, the last two functions are often shared with the other specialties, sometimes as a self-conscious effort at democratization of decision-making (hence the team) and sometimes because the other specialists disagree with the physician and modify or subvert his instructions if they think they can do so without getting into serious trouble.

However, all decisions involving patients' treatment and disposition require the formal approval of one or more physicians, and this fact accounts for much of the character of the program.

The medical model in action

The manner in which the various specialties are used and the time in a patient's program at which they are used depends to a considerable extent upon their utility in the eyes of the physicians. Thus, when a patient first comes on rehab, he will be scheduled for a "first review" based on evaluations prescribed by the physician to whom the patient has been assigned. The physician always expects an evaluation by the head nurse of the male or female ward even though he does not request one in writing. In addition, the physician prescribes evaluations by each of the other seven "disciplines" which he considers necessary. In the case of our sample of sixty patients, evaluations were prescribed with the following frequency:

Discipline	Number of Requests
Physical therapy	56
Social casework	56
Occupational therapy	55
Speech and hearing	38
Psychology	10
Vocational counseling	0
Social group work	0

The only cases in which physical therapists and social workers were not asked for evaluation were three cases in which the patients were not on the wards long enough for the initiation of such a request and one case in which the patient was on the ward solely for the purpose of securing an electric wheelchair. The five cases in which occupational therapists were not asked for evaluation included these four cases and one other in which the patient was transferred to the ward for some limited physical therapy only.

The above summary clearly reveals that for purposes of initial evaluation at least, the physician most often selects those specialties closely identified with improvement of the patient's physical health and the provision of welfare services.

While the choice of a social casework evaluation might, on the surface, seem to indicate a concern on the part of the physician with an appraisal of the patient's emotional or social problems, our observations indicate otherwise. In most cases, social casework on the rehab wards is primarily concerned with the processing of paper work necessary if the patient is to receive certain types of financial aid, prosthetic or assistive devices, and placement facilities outside of Farewell. (We will discuss the place of social work in the rehab program in more detail later in this chapter.)

The emphasis of the physicians on the patient's physical status is further revealed in the limited number of psychological evaluations requested. These are nearly always requested only if the patient has given evidence of being hard to manage or is suspected of suffering from brain damage. Although social group workers had been part of the team for more than a year at the time of our observations, they were never asked for an initial evaluation, and physicians were largely unaware of what their role might be or the actual work they did. Initial evaluation by a vocational counselor was never requested, largely as a result of the fact that most patients were either beyond the age of active employment or too disabled to work.

More of the disciplines got into the act at a later stage of the patient's career—evaluations after first review, actual counseling, or therapeutic work with the patient. For our sample of sixty, the distribution of such service is as shown.

The service of the group workers was almost entirely self-initiated. They took an interest in many of the patients, coun-

| | | Service Provided | |
| Name of | | Evaluation | Evaluation |
Specialty	None	Only	Plus
Physical therapy	4	8	48
Occupational therapy	5	20	35
Social casework	7	8	45
Social group work	18	21	21
Speech and hearing	22	32	6
Psychology	30	13	17
Vocational counseling	44	9	7

seled them, and made an effort to involve them in their group programs even though they were given no directives to work with any given patients. Like group workers, speech and hearing therapists enjoyed considerable autonomy in selecting cases for treatment. They carried out evaluations on request of the physicians, but the speech therapists themselves decided what patients should be placed on a given kind of speech therapy with almost no interference from the physicians, none of whom pretended to have any expertise in this area.

The information of the caseworker concerning the patient's social status was of importance to the physician in making disposition plans, and thus the caseworker's role in decision-making became more important in the latter part of the patient's stay on rehab. The OTs accepted over half the patients (in our sample) on their program, but in most cases dropped them in less than three months with no objections from the team physician. (It happens that in this hospital, psychology and vocational counseling resisted taking more cases and took them on only when pressed by other members of the team. Experience with these specialties is likely to be quite different in programs in which the specialists are striving to extend the scope of their services.)

The domination of the medical model is clearly reflected in the organization of the OT department. One shop was devoted to "functional therapy"—giving each patient on the program a series of exercises and tasks specifically designed to strengthen given muscles or to improve a given type of coordination or training skill in an ADL. The other shop was given over to "diversional activities" and provided projects for patients who requested them (rather than being assigned to them), e.g., weaving rugs, which would enable them to pass the time more creatively or enjoyably. The functional shop was obviously considered more important. The diversional shop was given over to the part-time direction of one OT, who was given this task because it was considered the least professional. The rest of the staff (sometimes numbering as many as six) were assigned to the functional program. Also, patients were evaluated only for functional therapy. The diversional program was regarded purely as a voluntary activity.

It is clear that the discipline most crucial to the physicians and thus most central to the rehab program is physical therapy. Despite the talk and writing about rehab as a team effort concerned with the total patient, to a great extent rehab is PT. When physicians, and often others, say a patient is not a good candidate for rehab, they almost always mean that he is not likely to benefit from further PT. When a physician decides that a patient is "too sick for rehab," he means that the patient is so sick that PT is contraindicated. The evaluations of the PTs dominated the decisions about the rehab programs of most patients—whether an active series of treatments was to be initiated, who were the best prospects for continued therapy, when therapy should be discontinued. "Progress" of a patient was mainly an evaluation of improvement in transfer and mobility, muscle strength and coordination, and the grosser aspects of self-care—aspects which were largely under the control of PT.

In large part, patients shared the physician's view of the role of the various specialties on rehab. When our sample of sixty was queried about their concept of rehab just before or shortly after they arrived on the ward, twenty-eight gave a usable response. (The rest had no preconception of rehab or were unable to communicate.) Only two of these made any mention of possible social, psychological, occupational, or educational benefits. The rest mentioned only improvement in physical function and ambulation, and—in the case of amputees—being fitted for a prosthetic leg.

We might expect the patients' concept of rehab to change in the direction of the professed rehab philosophy during their stay on the program. Although these conceptions did tend to become more differentiated, they still focused almost entirely on various forms of physical retraining plus the treatment of specific ailments by physicians. Of the forty-three patients in our sample for whom we were able to identify a definite conception of what rehab meant to them, only three put any stress on the social aspects of the program. They were all patients who had learned that they had progressive incurable diseases. Of the remaining seventeen, two could see no need for rehab, two consistently rejected all therapy, nine were too brain-damaged (usually with aphasia) or withdrawn to communicate with, and four were on rehab too short a time to develop a conception of rehab.

This does not mean that nearly one-third of all the patients on rehab at any given time lacked comprehension or appreciation of the therapeutic program. In general, patients who did not see the usefulness of the rehab program to themselves were likely to be discharged from the unit much sooner than others, so that they tended to be a considerably smaller group on the ward than they represented among the total number of admissions and discharges.

The amputees had the most clear-cut conception of rehab as it applied to them—obtaining a prosthetic leg and being trained to use it. Others stressed learning to walk, relearning activities of daily living, improving their strength and coordination, and obtaining special assistive devices. These are almost all PT functions, sometimes under the direction of physicians.

Even more convincing evidence of the central role of PT in

the eyes of the patients is the actions of patients when they had to make a choice of type of therapy. In three cases where patients thought that their PT and OT programs required too much of their time and energy, they all elected to go to PT and to drop OT. In another case a patient dropped her group work club activities because they interfered with her PT schedule. One patient who had his entire therapy program discontinued, tried hard to pull strings to get back on PT, but made no effort whatever to get back on his OT program. The sister of another patient transferred to a nursing unit because of acute illness and then moved to the nursing wards of rehab talked the staff into putting the patient back on PT, but did not try to get her on any other part of the program. In still another case where the speech therapy schedule conflicted with PT, the patient went to PT and simply did not show up for speech even though he was interested in pursuing the speech program.

Only one patient in our sample of sixty regularly continued his OT program while reducing his attendance at PT. This was a patient with a progressive disease who was rapidly getting weaker and who realized that he probably would not live much longer. We know of two other long-term patients outside of our sample of sixty who continued a regular OT program although they received little or no PT. Both of them were muscular dystrophy cases with no hope of improvement, but who could at best hope to avoid further deterioration.

Division of labor: experienced and inexperienced

The patient program was affected too by the fact that patient care tended to be left to the less experienced members of the staff. The senior physicians were men who were recognized specialists in their field. But they seldom examined or treated a patient at Farewell. This task was left almost entirely to foreign physicians fulfilling residency requirements. Every year there was a turnover in their ranks and a long-term patient might go through several physicians, all of them learning the rudiments of the specialty. OT received a crop of new graduates each year, most of whom would be ready for a "better job" by the following year. Although turnover in the other disciplines was not quite as drastic as in medicine and OT, the junior members of all the specialties were on the whole short-term employees.

The chiefs of the various specialties were much more stable. But with the exception of the physical therapy chief, they seldom worked with Farewell patients. Once or twice a year short courses for visiting students were conducted on the Farewell rehab unit. As part of this course, a few patients would be "staffed" so the students could see how a rehab team operates. On this occasion, all the chiefs (including the clinical director) evaluated one or two patients and presented a report at the meeting, often in an awkward manner because they were unaccustomed to the team procedures.

The staff may be thought of as being divided into a "demonstration team" made up of the most experienced and stable members of the staff and a "working team" made up largely of the less experienced and more transient members of the professional staff. During our stay at Farewell, only the PT chief had a place on both teams. This is not to say that the other chiefs rarely plied their trade with patients. Most of them did so, but not at Farewell. They did their clinical work at more prestigious and lucrative locations. They also spent much time in research, administration, teaching, and public relations.

Despite the fact that representatives of each specialty met as a team one or more times a week to discuss an agenda of cases, the treatment program was largely a fragmented affair—so much so that the more alert patients sometimes made an effort to coordinate the various aspects of the program, as we shall detail in Chapter 8. Each specialty cultivated its own garden in its own locations without day-to-day reference to the work of others.

There was little evidence of jurisdictional disputes. The psychologists and caseworkers did not clash over psychotherapy rights, because neither group had much time for it. The OTs concentrated on the finer movements of the hand and arm and on training in eating, dressing, and grooming. The PTs handled the grosser exercises for improving strength, range of motion, balance, and coordination, transfer and ambulation training, and fitting prosthetic legs, crutches, canes, and wheel-chairs. The division of labor between OT and PT is not one which is prescribed by their professional mandates. This ac-commodation is one that was worked out on the job at Fare-well before we got there. When we pointed it out to the therapists, they seemed surprised.

The most serious jurisdictional disputes (as well as the most frequent collaboration) occurred between the PTs and the doctors-in-training. The PTs often regarded the foreign resi-dents' judgment as faulty and would ignore, modify, or go be-yond their prescriptions. Although they probably "got away with" most of such actions, a resident would occasionally scold a PT for exceeding her formal authority.

Advantages and disadvantages of a nebulous role

The performance of the social caseworkers and social group workers neatly illustrates a number of the points made earlier in this chapter. We will therefore present their role on the rehab unit in more detail. We observed four caseworkers and three group workers, but they were not all there at the same time. All but one of them had a master's degree from a school of social work.

The tasks of the caseworkers are quite sharply defined by their medical superiors and co-workers from other specialties. The tasks of the group workers are scarcely defined at all.

These different expectations have their advantages and disadvantages.

THE CASEWORKER

As pointed out earlier, the team is primarily a medical team and the way in which the various specialties are used and the place in the rehabilitation program where they exert their influence depends to a considerable extent on how they serve the physicians.

The physicians use social casework information and services mainly to help determine and carry out the post-rehabilitation placement of the patients. Should the patient stay in an institution? Should he return to his family? Should he go to a rooming house or to a boarding home in which he will receive meals as well as shelter? In order to answer such questions, the physician must make some evaluation of the patient's life outside the hospital, both as it was before entering the hospital and as it potentially might be upon discharge. He must know something about the family relationships, the kinds of disabilities which a boarding home or rooming house will accept, the kind of financial arrangements which can be made for the support of the patient. This is the kind of information which the caseworker can supply. (At least she can supply more of it than can any of the other specialists.) In addition to supplying the information, the caseworker initiates and sometimes carries through on the actual processing of a discharge—making out forms to obtain housing, making applications for financial aid, arranging for casework follow-up.

The caseworker is also useful to the physician in explaining administrative procedures of public agencies such as the welfare department or the hospital department. These procedures are often crucial in getting prosthetic devices, wheelchairs, assistive appliances, home care, transfers and discharges, approval for job training. Some of the actual paper work involved in processing applications for therapeutic supplies and services is done by the caseworkers and they are expected to keep track of and expedite these orders—often a time-consuming task if pursued conscientiously. The caseworkers must also attend meetings at which the patients' cases are discussed so they may receive instructions from the physician about beginning the processing of orders or discharge as well as to give social work information about the patients' cases. In addition, the caseworker is expected to handle most of the outside contacts and inquiries from the patient's relatives and friends, lawyers, or other institutions and agencies.

Caseworkers on the rehab unit believe that their major function should be helping patients deal with their emotional and social problems. They should concern themselves with such matters as helping a patient accept his disability and his placement when he is moved off the rehab program, or making a patient's behavior more acceptable through a process of socializing him to conform more closely to behavior expected by the general public. To perform this function they may carry on a form of psychotherapy more usually referred to as "counseling." The caseworkers expect the patients to confide in them about emotional difficulties and interpersonal problems they are facing. One of the main modes of treatment are sessions, usually in the caseworker's office, in which these things are "talked through" in an effort to come to a solution which appears to deal with some important aspect of the patient's problem. Caseworkers realize, of course, that helping the patient with these problems often requires contacts with the family and friends and perhaps direct assistance with such things as housing, finances, or outside relationships. However, they believe that at least they should not become involved with the routine details of such contacts (e.g., placing prosthetic orders), but should be able to spend most of their time and energy directly with the patient's emotional problems.

The caseworker's ideal image of her professional role simply does not survive in this hospital setting. Instead of acting primarily as a counselor and therapist, she spends most of her time in the following ways:

Responsible for almost all contacts with family of patient.
Obtain information about patient.
Arrange meetings between physician and family members.
Search for family members whom the patient cannot contact.
Pass on information from physician to family.

Collect information about patient's background and present status from case records, interviews, home visits, and other sources. Obtain past medical records.

Deal with most outsiders interested in patient (except for medical consultations), including other institutions and agencies, family and friends, lawyers.

Process financial forms concerning patient and orders for prosthetic and assistive devices placed through the department of welfare, department of hospitals, and other agencies.

Keep track of orders and attempt to speed them up if delayed.

Provide information concerning patient's ability to live outside of hospital and make recommendations on discharge.

Arrange for placement in boarding house, rooming house, special camp or institution, patient's family if patient is to be discharged from hospital.
Arrange department of welfare aid on outside.
Arrange transportation.
Arrange trial visits.

Arrange for job training and placement (done only occasionally as a result of failure of vocational counseling service).

Discuss medical decisions on treatment and prognosis with patient (done occasionally by some workers as result of default by physicians).

Obtain clothing, recreational materials, and other items for patient.

Patients force upon the caseworker tasks which she does not consider appropriate. The patient needs clothes, he has to get a room to live in, he is not getting the kind of nursing service he should get, he wants a change in his medical therapy, he wants a wheelchair. He expects the caseworker to help him get these things. On the other hand, the great majority of patients do not see any need for counseling. They see their problems as things which require specific action to bring about some concrete result. Spending hours sitting in an office talking about the problems is likely to be regarded by them as an evasive operation. Quite frequently when such sessions are scheduled patients fail to show up for the appointment.

The physicians and other professional staff also supply the caseworker with tasks which the worker may consider inappropriate, but which she finds difficult to refuse. The physicians and some of the other professional workers may even consider the "counseling" as pointless as most of the patients do. When social workers are in short supply, there is likely to be even greater insistence by the physicians on getting specific, obvious, and concrete jobs done (e.g., collecting case histories on the patient and his family, ordering prosthetic devices, filling out forms for financial aid, making phone calls and writing letters to obtain a room for the patient to live in on the outside). Counseling is likely to be seen by patients and by other staff members as something you do only if you have enough time after carrying out the irreducible minimum of specific administrative functions. Thus, the caseworker spends a relatively large part of her time carrying out tasks which are thrust upon her and which she does not consider the proper job of a professional social worker.

THE GROUP WORKER

In contrast to the caseworkers, the group workers never have any definite major role on the team vis-à-vis the physician. They take part in the psychological management of the patients, but this is something that everybody on the team shares. At the first review and to some extent at later reviews of a patient's case, they report on the patient's social relationships with other patients. Usually little or nothing is done with this information by the physician in making his decisions about a patient's program. Although individual group workers may develop a good working relationship with individual physicians, and physicians may make use of the information they provide about the patients and may pay some attention to recommendations they make about patients' management, the specific aspects of group work as a therapeutic specialty are almost completely ignored by most physicians. This fact inevitably gives group work a marginal position on the rehab team.

The group workers, like the caseworkers, sometimes carry out functions which are generally thought of as belonging to other specialties, but the group workers are less likely to complain about it because these other functions are usually things which they like to do. For example, they engage in counseling patients just as caseworkers do, but they do it less systematically (e.g., they are less likely to make appointments to see patients in their offices and are more likely to have casual chats with patients in their cubicles or in the hallway). Also, they are not responsible for an assigned case load and can choose "interesting" cases to concentrate on. Some of their group programs border on group therapy although they are never called

that, but most of their efforts to manipulate group member-
ships and effect psychological changes in patients are made
through recreation-style programs.

The group worker's role conflicts are somewhat different
from those of the caseworker. Most of the other professional
specialists have an extremely nebulous notion about what a
group worker does and what patient service she is there for.
Since the physicians and other professional staff do not know
what specific tasks a group worker ought to carry out, they
seldom call upon her to perform given services for a patient or
to provide specific information about a patient's case. This
leaves the group worker relatively free from the constant
stream of "inappropriate" demands which the caseworker
suffers from.

The negative aspect of this situation is that group workers
receive little attention and little appreciation for what they do.
They have greater difficulty in getting the physician and other
staff members to perform what they consider important
services for the patients. Group workers repeatedly complain
that physicians ignore the social needs of the patient and deal
only with his medical problems. They complain that nurses
are not as helpful as they might be in organizing programs for
patients, or in helping patients to interact more effectively with
their fellows. Sometimes they find nurses obstructing group
activities when those activities seem to cause more work for
the nurses or upset the nursing routines. Physical therapists
and speech therapists have won recognition for their specific
therapeutic activities and can demand a place in the patients'
daily schedule. Group workers, on the other hand, must approach both nurses and patients in a more cautious fashion,
almost having to beg to be allowed to intrude their programs
into the ward routine.

Group work, in fact, tends to be regarded by the other pro-
fessions as a fringe benefit which can be readily reduced if
things get tough. The group workers must be careful not to

interfere with other forms of therapy or with routine nursing care. In contrast to other professional groups, they have to argue for equipment and space to carry on their programs.

The precarious position of the group work program was illustrated when the casework staff, which a year earlier had numbered three, was about to be reduced to one. It was generally agreed that one caseworker could not handle the entire unit. Therefore, the bulk of the case load which the resigning caseworker was leaving behind was divided between the two group workers, who consequently had to carry on their group work program on a part-time basis. Still later, an effort was made to convert the two group workers to full-time casework, at which point both resigned.

Thus, if the situation becomes critical and a choice must be made between maintaining a certain level of casework and reducing the group work program, or maintaining a given level of group work activities and reducing the casework tasks, the first of these alternatives is regarded as preferable. It is preferable because the controlling authorities (mainly the physicians) see casework as performing essential tasks in the processing of patients while the group work program is dismissed as a pleasant but unnecessary "extra."

THE CHOICE

Our observations illustrate two routes a social worker may follow in a public hospital setting: Make herself useful to the other professional staff and to the administrative operation by carrying out many routine chores that need to be done even though this often means reducing or even ignoring the therapeutic counseling role which she sees as central to her professional image (typical of the caseworkers on rehab); keep her job responsibilities so vague that no one can pin her down on what her tasks should be, but in this case she risks having her services dispensed with whenever the program is cut or the work load redistributed (typical of the group workers on rehab).

Of course, social workers prefer another alternative—educating the other professional staff and the patients about the proper role of social work and arranging that they be given only appropriate tasks. However, in view of the contradictory demands which public medical agencies make upon social workers and the relatively weak power position which social workers possess in such agencies, this goal will be difficult indeed to achieve.

Therapeutic-custodial dilemma

The ideology of the rehab movement emphasizes the "whole patient" approach. Ideally, everything done for or to the patient should be part of his total "therapy." Potentially, the patient's life may be viewed as one great rehab process subject to social control by a professional elite. In a program so conceived the burden of proof is on the patient to show that he does not need help from professionals in caring for given needs. Only a few patients with strong ties to the outside world are capable of such proof.*

Of course, the actual program we observed falls far short of this ideal conception. The professional staff is present only part of the time. They often fail to communicate with one another concerning a given patient. Some of them—particularly the foreign physicians—reject all or most of the ideology and often subvert its intent. Thus, in practice, patients are frequently left free of professional control. In addition, they find various dodges to avoid the controls of both the therapeutic and cus-

---

* A similar process occurs in mental hospitals when the conduct of the psychotherapist is taken as the model for other relationships in the hospital setting. See Alfred H. Stanton and Morris S. Schwartz, *The Mental Hospital* (Basic Books, 1954), pp. 146–151.

todial systems—a subject to which we will return in Chapter 8. The most unmistakable manner of escaping therapeutic controls is failure to cooperate with some or all aspects of their therapy program. This will cause the team to define them as "unmotivated" and they will soon be removed from the program and, when another place is found, from the rehab ward.

The emphasis of the professional rehab team is therapeutic rather than custodial. In fact, team members often direct caustic criticism toward the giant custodial institution in which their program is embedded and toward the ward staff whom they identify as agents of custodialism. Yet their day-to-day activities induce them to make contributions to the custodial operation. Their effort to make patients more independent is limited in practice largely to physical functioning per se. By continually planning for the patient, severely restricting his knowledge of his physical and social condition, and demanding that his life be subject to therapeutic control, inspection, and interpretation, the team contributes to the process of stripping the patient of moral and social identity and tends to return him to a position of childhood.

Even the physical independence toward which PT and OT strive simply makes patients somewhat more fit for custodial care. If the patients can care better for their own needs, they are less of a nursing burden. There is much emphasis on training in the use of a wheelchair—a mode of mobility for which Farewell Hospital, but not private residences or hotels, is admirably designed. Ambulation training is usually undertaken vigorously only when the team believes there is a place available for the patient in the community. A substantial portion of PT time is taken up with "maintenance therapy"—keeping a patient fit to live on a Farewell self-care unit—while he is waiting for orders for prosthetic or assistive devices to be processed or is awaiting transfer off the ward.

Almost all patients get caught in the public welfare system which usually seizes all their assets, often causes them to lose their residence, and interferes with help they might get from relatives and friends, to say nothing of subjecting them to what many of them regard as a degrading investigation. The rehab caseworkers do not approve of this process, in fact often inveigh against it, yet their position forces them to become collaborators in the investigation and the enforcement of welfare regulations. New caseworkers may want to do battle with the welfare system, especially those aspects which make it difficult for the patient to find a place to live in the community, but the extremely time-consuming process of arranging a community discharge for any case which is not cut-and-dried soon has most hard-pressed caseworkers agreeing that the typical rehab graduate may be just as well off on a Farewell self-care unit.

The vocational counselor puts most of his time and energy into getting contracts for the hospital-sheltered workshop—a pre-eminently custodial operation—and very little time to retraining and job-finding. Even the social group workers, the champions of the inmate against the "system," actually spend most of their working time helping patients adjust to their disability and to their life at Farewell.

Life in slow motion—   9
the therapeutic pace

The people who plan and direct a hospital rehabilitation program tend to think of the patient primarily as one of the units in that program and are concerned with his behavior insofar as it is related to that program. This, after all, is an active rehab program. The ongoing therapy is what sets this unit off from most of the other parts of this custodial institution. It is what makes rehab different from the rest of the hospital.

The active rehabilitation therapy program, however, makes up only a small part of the patients' lives. Just as in a psychiatric hospital the psychotherapy is for a select few and then only a few hours a week, rehab is for a small minority and for them limited to a narrow time span and a small part of any given day or week.

Rehab in small doses

During the period that we observed the selection clinic only 10 percent of those seen were transferred to the active rehabilitation unit. Of the sixty patients whose cases we followed, twenty were never placed on the therapy program at all or were dropped after a brief trial. At any given time, a substantial proportion of patients were not on the therapy program. During the week we made our systematic observations in therapy areas (an observer stationed in each therapy area kept a minute-by-minute record of patients present, the kind of therapy given them, and by whom), sixty out of eighty-five patients on the ward were actually receiving therapy—fifty, physical therapy; eleven, functional occupational therapy; seven, diversional occupational therapy; and two, in the sheltered workshop. (This breakdown adds up to more than sixty because some patients were on more than one therapy program.) The remaining twenty-five were not receiving therapy because they were: new patients who have not yet been put on the therapy program (this sometimes takes several weeks); temporarily off the program because of acute illness; amputees who are off the program while waiting for a prosthetic leg or for adjustment of prostheses (this may take several months); patients whose program was discontinued when they were slated for transfer or discharge (sometimes a lapse of several months from decision to actual discharge); patients who are being carried on the rehab unit for "social reasons"—for example, some of the young adults and muscular dystrophy cases for whom rehab serves as a custodial unit.

If we consider only the fifty patients receiving PT, the time in the gyms, if distributed evenly among them, would amount to about one hour per day of which approximately fifteen minutes would consist of direct treatment by the PT staff, twenty minutes of self-treatment (for example, exercising oneself with lifting weights, practicing crutch walking by oneself), or in passive treatment (for example, sandbags left in position to stretch the knee; patient left in a vertical position on the tilt table). The remainder of the hour would be spent waiting one's turn.

In OT functional therapy, if we consider only the eleven patients actually on the program, the time in the shop, if distributed evenly among them, would amount to about one hour each, of which again about fifteen minutes would consist of direct attention from an OT staff member, about forty minutes spent working by oneself, and the remaining period in waiting time. For the OT diversional shop, if we consider only the seven actually on the program, the time distributed evenly among them would again amount to about one hour for each, which would include about one minute's attention from the staff, and the rest of the time working by oneself. We will disregard the sheltered workshop from further consideration because of the very small number of rehab patients who were on this program at the time. The following shows the use of the therapies by the patients observed:

	PT	Functional OT	Diversionary OT
Number of patients (out of 85)	50	11	7
Mean time in therapy area	60 min.	60 min.	60 min.
Mean time treated by staff	15 min.	15 min.	1 min.
Mean time in passive or self-treatment	20 min.	40 min.	59 min.
Waiting time	25 min.	5 min.	—

But therapy time is not equally distributed among the patients on the program. Nine patients were receiving physical therapy more than an hour a day, five were receiving functional occupational therapy more than an hour a day. This means other patients were receiving less than that amount of time. Even for the few receiving the longer periods of therapy, the one to two hours a day made up only a small fraction of their total day. And on weekends and the many holidays, there was no program at all.

This is not to argue that all patients would necessarily benefit from spending much more of their time on PT or OT, but only to point out that the formal therapy takes up a very small part of the patients' waking hours. It is also clear that the amount of therapy is determined largely by staff schedules. A physician's recommendation to expand a patient's program is sometimes not carried out or a patient's therapy is delayed because the therapists' schedules are full at the time. Again, the situation is similar to the psychiatric hospital where the therapists have only a limited number of hours per day for psychotherapy.

The waiting game

It is not only the small doses of therapy each day or week which may stretch out the patient's stay in the rehab program. Much of the delay is simply a matter of waiting for something to happen.

Complex bureaucracies serving a clientele maintain procedures designed to keep the staff from being overworked and to make sure none of the clients is given anything he is not entitled to. Where the clientele consists of the lowly and unwanted, these restraints on service apply with even greater force because the clients lack the bargaining power to effectively press for more expeditious decisions and actions. In the case of the rehab program, certain external factors, such as the shortage of housing, slow up the process still further.

Patients coming to Farewell Hospital have often spent considerable time in other institutions waiting for decisions to be made on their cases. We will not present the details on previous institutional stay because our information is scattered and not very reliable in some cases—records are notoriously incomplete and inaccurate on this point. However, in those cases where we had confidence in the information, most patients had spent at least four months in other institutions, some over a year. A psychologist who tried to find a sample of new patients who had spent less than three months in other hospitals before coming to Farewell soon gave up because he found so few cases. If patients come to rehab by way of the admission wards and selection clinic, they will have spent from one week to two months waiting on the admission wards before being moved to rehab (the median is about three weeks).

After getting to rehab, they will spend from one to three weeks being evaluated and waiting for the first team meeting. This length of time simply for an initial evaluation is long by general hospital standards, but short in comparison to the pace that patients must become accustomed to in this hospital. Of the 85 percent of the patients coming to rehab who at least get started on the therapy program, some begin therapy even before they have their first team meeting, most others immediately after. The few who have to wait several weeks to get on therapy are usually those who have some complicating disorder which has to be checked so as to ensure that the exercises and training are appropriate and safe.

Another source of delay is the time consumed obtaining prostheses and assistive devices. The great majority of patients are on department of welfare aid, and any assistive devices obtained for them must be ordered and approved by this department. Approved orders are referred to the purchasing department, which then places the order with a contractor or obtains bids. Finally, the dealer in these devices himself must process the order, and, in some cases, actually make the device before it can be delivered. The fact that quality considerations were usually ignored in bidding for contracts meant that the devices delivered were frequently inadequate and either had to be rejected—thus waiting for the order to be processed again—or returned for adjustments, sometimes repeatedly. Such re- orders or adjustments, of course, added to the waiting time.

Although prosthetic legs for amputees in our sample were always ordered within a month or two after the patients' first team meeting, it took from three to eight months after the physicians' prescriptions for the prosthetic legs to be delivered and final adjustments made so that the patients could be trained in their use (median was four months). Another one to ten months elapsed between the time of final adjustment of the prosthetic legs and the time of discharge from rehab (me- dian was four and one-half months). An extreme case is that of Harvey Coots, who waited for eight months after the order had been placed to get a below-knee prosthesis, which he learned to use within a few weeks without any training at all. In other words, almost all of his time on rehab consisted simply of waiting. The proportion is not as great in most cases, but for many patients, especially the amputees, it is a substantial portion of their time on rehab.

An amputee who does not have to rely on the department of welfare and has a home outside of the hospital need not wait at Farewell Hospital during the period of time spent making the prosthetic leg, but can go home until the prosthesis is ready and then return to rehab for training. This was done by Albert Hetherton, who entered rehab with a leg already de- livered and properly adjusted, received six weeks of training, became ambulatory, and returned to his home (compared with the median of four and one-half months for all patients). A similar procedure was followed by Gloria Crane, who went home after the preliminary work on the stumps of her legs was completed and returned to Farewell when the prosthetic legs were ready. Because she was a bilateral amputee with some complications in one stump, the process took about four and one-half months, but this was still less time than that required of other patients with similar problems.

Another device which is ordered for many patients is a wheelchair. Wheelchairs differ from prosthetic legs in that they usually do not have to be made to order. One of several basic designs can have attachments readily added according to the physician's prescription. Thus a factory-made end product can be ready shortly after an order has been placed. However, for department of welfare cases even these orders take a substantial period of time to process. The time from the first team meeting to the time of ordering a wheelchair varied from zero (that is, a wheelchair decided upon at the first team meeting and ordered the next day) to twelve and one-half months (median was one month). Those cases that took considerably more time than the median almost always resulted from the staff's uncertainty about the patient's need for a wheelchair and the subsequent trial period in which an attempt was made to ambulate the patient before deciding whether the wheelchair should be ordered.

Twelve of the fifteen orders for wheelchairs placed through the department of welfare were completed during our period of observation. The time from the ordering of the chair to its delivery varied from two months to seven and one-half months (median was five months). In the case of two patients, the wheelchair was paid for by their families and the usual complex process of ordering through the welfare department was avoided. In one of these two cases the chair was delivered seven days after the order was placed, and in the other case, fifteen days later. These periods of time probably represent the time that it takes the dealer to handle the order. The remainder of the five months required in other cases represents the administrative processes of the public agencies involved.

Rehab staff who were upset by these delays (usually newer staff members who have not become used to the standard pace yet) sometimes made an effort to speed up the process, but we did not observe any great success in their efforts. One social worker made a particular effort to expedite the wheelchair of Allen Putnam by calling people whom she knew in the department of welfare and arguing that the case was an urgent one. Still it took three and one-half months from the time of her call before Putnam received his wheelchair.

Sometimes the ordering of the wheelchair was delayed by a change in treatment plans. When the original prognosis was that a patient would learn to walk, the physician did not feel justified in ordering a wheelchair right away. After the therapy had continued for some time and the patient did not make the expected gains, the staff might decide that he needed a wheelchair (or some other device) after all, and eventually place an order quite a long time after the patient has come on rehab. Why, one may ask, didn't the staff order a wheelchair early in the patient's stay in case he might need it later and simply return the chair (or use it for another patient) if the patient for whom it was ordered learned to walk? In fact, the staff occasionally did this, but they were then taking other risks. If the patient proved to need a walker (supportive frame on wheels used as partial support while walking) or crutches or some other device instead of a wheelchair, it might be difficult to get the second order approved because money had been "wasted" on the patient for the unnecessary first order. Also, a device ordered for one patient cannot be given to another—even if this is a standard product—but must be returned to the welfare department. That is, the treatment staff is not permitted to stockpile equipment (although they surreptitiously manage to do so on a limited scale), but must go through the ordering process for each patient. Thus, the official welfare policies had the effect of encouraging the staff to put off placing orders until they were "sure" of the outcome and exactly what the patient will need in the end.

Other appliances and mechanical aids were ordered less frequently than wheelchairs, but these also could take a long time to obtain. A walker ordered for a patient in our sample took five and one-half months to be delivered. Of six brace orders for patients in our sample, the time from the first team meeting to placing the order ranged from eight days to seven months, with a median of about four months. The time from placing the order to the delivery of the brace varied from fourteen days to seven months, with a median of about five months. Contrast this with the case of Carlos José, whose family paid for the brace and thus avoided the department of welfare purchasing procedure. In this case the brace was delivered in less than one week.

Of course, waiting for a mechanical aid to be delivered does not always delay therapy because some aspects of therapy can go on which do not rely on this appliance. Also, waiting for wheelchairs and walkers does not necessarily hold up discharge because—once the items have been approved by welfare—the patient may be discharged from rehab and return to the prosthetic clinic when delivery is made. But often some part of the patient's program must be delayed and the patient must be kept on rehab for a time simply in order to be eligible for the appliance. The career of Samuel Nash on rehab is one of the more "pure cases" of such administrative delay. Nash never had any team meetings and was never placed on a physical therapy program because the staff did not consider him a "real rehab patient." He had been "temporarily" transferred to the rehab unit to obtain a motorized wheelchair. He spent almost a year on rehab. Actually, he initially obtained the wheelchair somewhat more quickly than most patients because he was given an old used chair which was already on hand. This plan for quick action backfired because the chair broke down repeatedly, and months of time were consumed waiting for repairs and new parts, some of which had to be obtained through the usual welfare procedures. There was further delay in transferring him back to a medical ward.

Another time-consuming process is that of discharge to the community and inter-ward transfer. In our sample we have definite information on the final decision made by the staff (statements in team meeting, physicians' notes, statements by social worker) to transfer a patient to another Farewell ward in twenty-seven cases. The time from the staff's final decision to make such a transfer to the actual carrying out of the transfer varied from six days to nine months (median was one and one-half months).

In the case of patients discharged to the community, we have definite information on the final staff plans in fourteen cases. The time from the final staff decision to discharge the patient to the community until the time of actual discharge ranged from zero (in one case where discharge took place immediately after the decision was made) to four and one-half months, with a median of one and one-half months. Here again, much of the processing must be done through welfare, which must locate and approve the patient's housing if the patient is to receive welfare aid on the outside.

The patient may remain on rehab for some time after all therapy has been canceled. Of those transferred to other Farewell wards, we have information on the time that therapy programs stopped for twenty-three in our sample. The amount of time from the period that therapy stopped to the time that the patient was transferred off rehab ranges from zero (that is, the patient received therapy right up to the time of transfer) to nine months, with a median of about one month.

Of those discharged to the community, fourteen out of eighteen received physical therapy until the time of their discharge. The remaining four had periods of time off therapy up to as much as five and one-half months. In effect, patients who are kept on rehab after they have reached their "maximum" or "plateau" and have their therapy program discontinued are simply boarders on the rehab unit, much as hundreds of others are boarders on other Farewell units, especially in the self-care building. The difference is that most of the custodial units are intended to function as such highly protective boarding homes, whereas rehab is supposed to have a special therapeutic place in the hospital structure. But these patients, though they fill up rehab beds without being on the rehab program, do not particularly trouble the therapists, except the physicians and nurses who must continue to tend to their variety of ills so long as they are there.

[In passing, it is interesting to note how rehab personnel use "maximum" or "reaching a plateau" to indicate the level of physical function at which a patient is not likely to improve any further. Thus, when a patient reaches maximum, rehab therapy can do no more for him and he may be dropped from the therapy program or, in some cases, continued for "maintenance"—that is, to keep the patient from regressing to a more dependent level.

Maximum is a vague concept because it is almost always used without specifying the conditions under which the lack of further progress may be expected. Thus, Joe McCormick, who was considered to have reached his maximum at a nonambulatory level while on rehab, has succeeded in walking on the street with a cane and with some help from his wife since he has been discharged. Herbert Witton was transferred to a nursing unit still largely dependent in self-care and regarded as incapable of further improvement after he had refused to cooperate in a therapy program. Once off rehab and without any further program in PT or self-care training, he improved sufficiently in self-care in a half-year's time to be considered eligible for transfer to a self-care custodial ward.

Marcia Brant was regarded as having "reached a plateau" according to a physician's note in October, at which time she was ambulatory only with considerable assistance from a walker and was still partly dependent in self-care. Physical therapists continued to work with her and by February of the following year they had her walking—although shakily—with a cane and maintained they could improve her walking still further and make it safer with more training.

The temptation to label a patient "maximum" when one wants to get rid of him for any reason is no doubt great. One must recognize that such labeling is not an objective or readily definable point in a patient's therapeutic development, but only a very rough and frequently mistaken prognosis about the patient's physical function. Different staff members sometimes disagree about when maximum has been reached by a given patient. Patients are sometimes unwilling to accept staff judgment about when they have reached their maximum, and if sufficiently insistent, may induce the staff to continue them on therapy.]

Therapists, especially physical therapists, are annoyed by patients who are being carried as boarders, but who are also continued on PT by a physician's prescription. The PTs may maintain that such patients do not need therapy, cannot benefit from therapy, or are past the point where they can get any good out of therapy. PTs feel that they are being asked to work with such patients simply because the patients are there, and they see this as a waste of time and effort which might be better spent with some other patient who still has potential for improvement.

When a patient is moved off rehab for a diagnostic work-up (a series of laboratory tests) or for special treatment, he may have a difficult time getting back on rehab and thus his program will be stretched out further. When Allen Putnam was transferred to another hospital for a neurological examination, he was kept there from two to three weeks after all the diagnostic examinations had been concluded. When he was returned to Farewell, he was placed on the admission ward instead of being directly readmitted to rehab as the physicians had originally ordered. It was not until he had lain around the admitting ward for ten days and his wife made inquiries of the rehab physicians that he was finally transferred back to rehab.

The case of Mary Anne Kraft is an even more extreme illustration of this type of delay. It also exemplifies the belief of many patients that they are not free to leave the hospital without official approval, even if they are ready and have a housing accommodation.

Thirteen days after coming on rehab, Miss Kraft had an orthopedic consultation and hip surgery was advised. Two days later she was transferred to a medical unit for treatment of anemia and further diagnosis. While she was on this ward, a medical resident asked her to sign an authorization for hip surgery. She refused because (she said) she had been advised against this by an outside physician she trusted more and because no information on her diagnostic test results or any other aspect of her case had ever been discussed with her during her stay at Farewell. A month after she had been transferred to the medical unit, a physician's note in her chart stated that she could be returned to rehab. There were no more physicians' notes written on her case for the next seven weeks. Nine weeks after the note was written, she was returned to rehab. She was now scheduled for her first team meeting and a decision was reached to train her to use crutches and plan for community discharge. Two months later she had her second team meeting. The staff then decided to have her ambulate in a walker. They noted that Miss Kraft's family was maintaining her apartment, which placed her in a far better position to be discharged than the vast majority of patients. The team physician directed that she be scheduled for another team meeting in four weeks. Actually, her third team meeting did not occur for three and one-half months. The decision was to continue the same therapy. No mention was made of discharge even though this was labeled a discharge meeting. Her condition showed no further improvement, so there was no point in her staying longer. No action was taken. Three weeks after her third team meeting she learned that her social worker was planning a long vacation and had taken no steps to arrange her discharge. Her efforts to press for discharge failed again. Another month and one-half went by. Then she received a letter from her brother in which he threatened to stop paying for her apartment if she did not get out of the hospital and return to her apartment promptly. She showed this letter to the staff and was discharged a few days later. The researchers suspect that the letter was a product of collusion—that is, that Miss Kraft asked her brother to send her an ultimatum so she could use it to prod the staff into action. Total time on rehab for Mary Anne Kraft: twelve months, twenty-two days. Change in physical function: virtually none.

Still other things hold up progress on certain cases. For example, in the case of patients who are unable to get to the therapy areas on their own, therapy sessions are sometimes skipped because the hospital messenger service fails to bring the patient to the therapy area when scheduled. In still other cases, tests and consultations requested by the rehab staff physicians may take a long time to be performed. The difficulties in having an intravenous polygram (IVP) performed on John Green may have been exceptionally great, but yet the case illustrates a not uncommon feeling about the speed with which things may be expected to be carried out at Farewell Hospital.

The first report we find of an intravenous polygram being requested on Green was on August 23. The next record appears on December 13 of the same year when Green's ward physician wrote a note that the IVP was being requested for the third time. It is not clear what happened to the second request or whether the August 23 was the second request and the first request was not recorded. On March 28 of the following year another resident who had taken over the case wrote "IVP requested again!" The test was finally carried out two days later. Thus there was a delay of at least seven months from the initial request to the actual carrying out of the order for this test, one which may be of some importance in the case of a quadriplegic with urinary difficulties. Not only is the amount of the delay important, but so is the apparent equanimity with which the delay is accepted by the medical residents on the rehab unit. When their request for a test or consultation is not carried out, they seem to be willing to wait several months before asking again. This illustrates nicely the pace at which they expect the hospital as a whole to operate. In cases like this, they seldom, if ever, make any complaints about the fact that the requests are not being expeditiously handled. All one observes is a trace of annoyance which shows up as an exclamation point in the physician's progress notes as the request is made for the fourth time.

Reducing the wait

Outside of such specific delays, what about the pace of the program as a whole? This is very difficult to define. Some patients cannot be moved along at a very fast pace and for some perhaps a half hour a day PT is all that is beneficial. Some, especially those with a recent "stroke," must await a degree of spontaneous recovery—analogous to maturation in a child—before training in certain skills can profitably be undertaken, although other types of therapy must be begun on these patients to prevent potentially irreversible damage, such as contractures and muscle atrophy.

However, it is still clear—in fact, the therapists often state—that more intensive therapy with certain patients would bring them to their maximum capacity sooner and thus make it possible to get them off the rehab unit sooner. Physicians sometimes prescribe "intensive"—in effect, speeded up—therapy in special cases. Albert Hetherton was paying his own way and was anxious to work very hard and get the training in the use of a prosthesis rapidly so as to return home. The staff accommodated him by giving him several long periods of intensive training each day, succeeded in making him ambulatory and getting him out of the hospital in six weeks, about one-third the median time for amputees to go through the usual cycle of training and discharge after receiving a prosthetic leg through the department of welfare. Loretta Gump was also put on such an intensive program by the physicians and PTs when she first came because they saw a good possibility of making her independently ambulatory and discharging her to the community in a short time. It was only when the possibility of community discharge became very unlikely that the pace of the therapy was greatly reduced.

In general, the more seriously affected hemiplegics are not regarded as good candidates for intensive therapy and rapid discharge to the community, and thus they are not often given such intensive programs. Carlos José is a clear-cut exception and his timetable shows that he benefited from the intensive program of the staff as well as his own forcing of exercise and training.

José benefited not only from an intensive therapy program and by training himself outside the therapy area; he also benefited from the fact that his family paid for the brace and thus cut out the waiting time which might have delayed his discharge for months. When the brace needed some minor adjustment, rather than returning it to the physicians (he had heard from other patients that such adjustments often take weeks), he arranged to have someone take him to the hospital machine shop where he found a Spanish-speaking workman (José is Puerto Rican) who was willing to use the machine-shop tools to make this adjustment for him.

José's entire program on rehab took four and one-half months and made him independently ambulatory and independent in self-care. The median for other hemiplegics in our sample who were placed on a physical therapy program and were discharged to the community or to a nursing home was about eight months, and all were on rehab considerably longer than José.

This is not to say that every patient who received a very intensive program from the therapists succeeded in getting out sooner than the average. Several young adults received very intensive programs and did not seem to benefit much by them. However, they usually had no place to go on the outside and thus were doomed to stay in the hospital anyway. Since the rehab staff were reluctant to place these young adults on custodial wards with large concentrations of seriously disabled aged patients, they were likely to spend long stretches of time on the rehab unit. There seems no doubt, however, that in some of the cases where intensive application of therapy and a special effort at placement were made by the staff, a substantially shorter period on the rehab unit resulted.

In some other cases, the pace of therapy tended to be slower than average. These were usually patients with poor prognoses who did nothing to urge the staff to move them along faster and probably would have had no chance for community discharge. They may possibly have been ready for transfer to another ward sooner if the pace of therapy had been speeded up.

The conference system of teams of cooperating specialists may also contribute to slowing the pace of the program from the viewpoint of the individual patient. Certainly that is the effect of such a system in mental hospitals and tuberculosis hospitals and seems to be so on the rehab unit. When decisions on a case are at an impasse—e.g., uncertainty or disagreement or external blocks on placement of a patient—the standard practice is to postpone the decision to another meeting. Sometimes the purpose of this later discussion is to include further information gathered by social workers, the accumulation of more test information by physicians, or information about the potentiality of the patient as a result of further PT or OT training. However, the process of getting this information may take up only part of the time in which the discussion has been postponed. On the other hand, in some cases the scheduling of another team meeting speeds the gathering of information by forcing the responsible staff member to meet a deadline.

With the team decision-making system, this process of putting off decisions is necessary. Just the matter of getting all these different specialists together to discuss the case is a major scheduling problem and must ordinarily be limited to rather infrequent set times when any given case must compete with other urgent cases. A difficult discharge case such as Samuel James had four different discharge meetings over a period of more than a year before he was finally discharged.

Not every decision about a patient's treatment and placement must wait for a team meeting. Many decisions are made outside of team meetings, including some which, according to formal procedure, are supposed to be made only at a team meeting. Decision-making on the part of single individuals or conferences between two individuals (for example, between physician and PT, between physician and social worker) often represent a reaction on the part of staff to the frustration of having to wait for a team meeting to get some new action started on a given case. However, this practice of bypassing other team members raises problems of its own and therefore must be used with caution.

The chronic pace

Every work group must control the demands made upon its time. This is partially done by extending the work over time and refusing to allow the urgencies of those who are served to intrude upon one's life. Every complex of institutional procedures tends to sacrifice the time and convenience of the inmate for the sake of avoiding the disruption of the pace at which the institution is designed to operate.

The differences which may be found between total institutions on this score is one of degree, though the degree of difference in some cases may be rather great. Whereas a general hospital patient may have his discharge delayed one day because the laboratory technician does not want to work overtime or a physician cannot conveniently make a call, the rehab patient may have his discharge delayed for weeks or months because the prosthetic order is slow in being processed, the therapy staff cannot expand its program, or the department of welfare does not have appropriate housing available.

The chronic custodial treatment institution, in comparison with a short-term treatment institution, seems like a study in slow motion. Even the staff of several years' experience are often misled about the pace at which their program moves. Their predictions about when a patient will reach a given point in his program almost always fall short. "Transfer in two weeks" becomes three months. "Have him ambulatory in two months" becomes six months. "Will get him into a furnished room in one month" turns out to take four months. "Will have information from his consultation next week" ends up coming two months later. It is something the staff becomes accustomed to and after a while they notice only the extreme cases—the wheelchairs that take eight months for delivery instead of the usual five months. It is something the patients become accustomed to also, but often with much more bitterness.

Inmate tacks: coming to terms with the system 7

"Adjusting" to a situation usually means one wishes the situation did not exist but there is no immediate possibility of escape. It is safe to say that almost all Farewell inmates consider themselves in such a position.

"Adjustment" may be approached from a number of angles. There is the manipulation of one's personality in relation to one's surroundings. This approach will not be used in this book since we did not direct our inquiry in this direction. There is the use of various dodges to find a better life in the crevices of the formal structure. This will be dealt with in some detail in Chapter 8. There is also the matter of relating to the structure itself—positively, negatively, tangentially. This aspect will be the main focus of this chapter.

The patient as an institutional inmate

The rehab patients are not only the patients of a medical organization and the charges of a personal care service, but are also the inmates of what approximates an ideal total institution. Erving Goffman specifies the characteristics of such an institution as follows:

> First, all aspects of life are conducted in the same place and under the same single authority. Second, each phase of the member's daily activity is carried on in the immediate company of a large batch of others, all of whom are treated alike and required to do the same thing together. Third, all phases of the day's activities are tightly scheduled, with one activity leading at a prearranged time into the next, the whole sequence of activities being imposed from above by a system of explicit formal rulings and a body of officials. Finally, the various enforced activities are brought together into a single rational plan purportedly designed to fulfill the official aims of the institution.
>
> . . . there is a basic split between a large managed group, conveniently called inmates, and a small supervisory staff. Inmates typically live in the institution and have restricted contact with the world outside the walls; staff often operate on an eight-hour day and are socially integrated into the outside world. Each grouping tends to conceive of the other in terms of narrow hostile stereotypes, staff often seeing inmates as bitter, secretive, and untrustworthy, while inmates often see staff as condescending, highhanded, and mean. Staff tends to feel superior and righteous; inmates tend, in some ways at least, to feel inferior, weak, blameworthy, and guilty.*

Of course, at Farewell Hospital the scheduling of an in-

*Erving Goffman, *Asylums* (Garden City, N.Y.: Doubleday, 1961), pp. 6–7. Conceptually, this chapter is based largely on one of the essays in this book: "On the Characteristics of Total Institutions," pp. 12–60.

mate's activities is not nearly as tight as in a prison, and this has some important consequences to be mentioned later. There are also more differences of opinion among staff about the aims of the institution than we usually find in a prison and therefore less consistency in the over-all plan of operation. Thus, there is a greater variety of staff stereotypes about patients than in a more completely total institution and the patient has a choice of more niches to move into and a greater range of staff groups to ally himself with than is usually found in a prison situation. The implications of this are also taken up in other parts of this report.

One aspect of total institutions which is found to a somewhat diluted degree at Farewell is the induction procedure in which a patient is classified and assigned through a process of case-history documentation, physical examination, the issue of clothing, instruction in the rules and procedures and expectations of the hospital, and assignment to quarters. This is a process of codifying and categorizing a newcomer to fit the institutional program. His unique characteristics and his own desires tend to be treated as inconsequential or even disturbing to the total program.

The inmate is permitted little in the way of his own possessions. Housekeeping is difficult. There is not much room to store things and theft is common. Most of the things inmates use and, for many, most of the clothes they wear, belong to the institution. Institutional issue is the usual coarse, ill-suited variety and much the same for all inmates.

The round of life is one that tends to make the inmates' time and effort seem worthless. On rehab, for example, the slow pace of the therapeutic program (a little each day), the long delays in getting equipment and appliances, the long wait for community placement in case of discharges, the weeks and months spent on another ward waiting to be returned to rehab after receiving some specialized medical treatment, and many other instances of frittering away the inmates' time might be cited.

The inmate finds that many different staff members and other institutional authorities garner information about him and communicate it to other people, often recording this information in documents open to a variety of people. This includes information about the patient's past life, details of his present physical and psychological disabilities, embarrassing events in his daily life, and sometimes a diagnosis of his psyche. He learns that such information may be used against him in making treatment and discharge decisions. Thus, the department of welfare has full access to all records kept on him and may use this information to his disadvantage. His incoming mail may be opened—certainly not routinely as in prisons, but often enough to worry some patients and to cause them to have outgoing letters which are critical of hospital procedures smuggled out of the hospital by visitors to be deposited in a mailbox off the grounds. (We have no evidence of outgoing mail being opened by the staff, but patients fear that it is.) Lockers and bedside tables may be inspected at any time by hospital employees. Such garnering and communication of information about the patient is regarded as proper and standard procedure by the staff, and if the staff is not well informed about a given patient, they regard this as a defect in their system rather than as a protection of the privacy of the inmate.

The inmate finds that spheres of activity cannot be kept separate as they often were in his pre-institutional world. His reputation in one sphere of activity directly affects his reputation in other spheres throughout the institution. His performance on the ward, as well as his performance in the therapy sessions, affects the judgment of the therapists about his abilities. In fact, for rehab to be considered successful, it is regarded as essential for the inmate's performance outside of the therapy sessions to be affected. That is, the physical tasks he has apparently learned in therapy sessions are not considered really learned if the patient is not able to perform equally well in his life on the ward. But from the viewpoint of some patients, who may simply be trying to make a good impression so that they are left alone to enjoy themselves, this overlap of spheres of behavior represents an invasion of the privacy which they knew earlier.

The patient finds that his needs for service are defined by the employees, not by himself. Patients frequently believe that they require and are entitled to certain services or certain supplies or treatment which the staff, for whatever reason, does not want to give at that time. The patient may thus be placed in a position where he has to ask repeatedly for something he believes he needs and is entitled to. The complaints may earn him a bawling out and perhaps poorer service. A bad reputation among one specialty group or one sphere of activity may soon get around to other groups and spheres and earn the patient a general reputation as a troublemaker.

However, no matter what the environmental pressures may be, the inmate must make some kind of adaptation to the institutional complex where he lives so long as he remains there. On the basis of examples from concentration camps, prisons, mental hospitals, military camps, merchant ships, and other more or less totally controlled institutions, Goffman derives four "tacks" which an inmate may take.

1. *Situational withdrawal.* "The inmate withdraws apparent attention from everything except events immediately around his body and sees these in a perspective not employed by others present."

2. *Intransigent line.* "The inmate intentionally challenges the institution by flagrantly refusing to cooperate with staff. . . . Although some prisoners of war have been known to take a staunchly intransigent stance throughout their incarceration, intransigence is typically a temporary and initial phase of reaction, with the inmate shifting to situational withdrawal or some other line of adaptation."

3. *Colonization.* "The sampling of the outside world provided by the establishment is taken by the inmate as the whole, and a stable, relatively contented existence is built up out of the maximum satisfactions procurable within the institution. Experience

of the outside world is used as a point of reference to demonstrate the desirability of life on the inside, and the usual tension between the two worlds is markedly reduced. . . . Colonizers may feel obliged to deny their satisfaction with the institution, if only to sustain a counter-mores supporting inmate solidarity. They may find it necessary to mess up just prior to their slated discharge to provide themselves with an apparently involuntary basis for continued incarceration."

4. *Conversion.* "The inmate appears to take over the official or staff view of himself and tries to act out the role of the perfect inmate. While the colonized inmate builds as much of a free community for himself as possible by using the limited facilities available, the convert takes a more disciplined, moralistic, monochromatic line, presenting himself as someone whose institutional enthusiasm is always at the disposal of the staff."*

Inmate tacks on rehab

ESCAPE

When Goffman spoke of situational withdrawal, he used the mental hospital as a primary model and concentrated on various forms of psychological withdrawal—a cutting off of oneself from interaction with one's immediate surroundings. We find some of this on rehab, though it is probably much more common on many of the other hospital wards where one can find large numbers of patients sitting for long periods in wheelchairs or benches in a thickly populated day room, apparently not noticing or reacting to what is going on around them. This kind of withdrawal is sometimes a result of serious brain damage which depresses the patient's reactivity—some rehab patients will sit in a busy area and sleep off and on for long periods. However, a more common type of escape on rehab among those who are physically able is bodily removal from areas where most interaction with the staff takes place. Such a patient goes off by himself for long periods of time, some-

* *Ibid.,* pp. 61–64.

times for almost the entire day. Some patients go out-of-doors and move away from the immediate hospital area to the more remote corners of the grounds. Some sit in corridors by themselves, sometimes just staring out of the window, sometimes with eyes closed.

A patient following the escape pattern may or may not show up for therapy. Such patients are often removed from the therapy program for a long time while still on rehab, partly because the therapists have so much difficulty getting them to attend their sessions. The escape pattern is likely to be regarded as a form of psychopathology by the staff and as a most unhopeful sign for rehabilitation. The nursing staff usually makes no effort to hold such patients on the ward and are often glad to get rid of them for most of the day, since these patients are likely to engage in disturbing behavior if forced to stay in the midst of other people.

Of course, one form of escape from the situation is to leave the hospital against advice (and two of our sample of sixty did this), but this does not represent a common pattern of inmate life.

Proportionately, an escape pattern is relatively frequent among the rehab population. If we include one patient who committed suicide (and suicide may be regarded as the ultimate form of escape from a situation), at least ten of our sample of sixty—eight of them men—fit the extreme form of withdrawal quite closely.

ATTACK

Open attack on the staff or flagrant refusal to cooperate, although by no means an infrequent experience in the day's work of the staff, tends to be a relatively rare event in the career of a given patient. Evading or undermining the treatment program or work procedures is more likely to be hidden and underhanded and will elicit some explanation or apology if detected. Abusive attacks on the staff are usually avoided even when the patient feels extremely bitter about being put upon. Of our sixty patients, one refused to observe an important part of the ward routine (staying out of his bed during the day) as soon as he came on the ward and lasted only about five hours on rehab. We learned of similar intransigence on his part later on in other wards (e.g., refusing to exchange wheelchairs when asked by a doctor and nurses), but we did not observe him closely over a period of time.

Another patient complained loudly day after day on the ward, especially early in the night, disturbing both ward staff and other patients. She also would not cooperate with procedures in the physical therapy gym. Her program was cut short and she was transferred soon after. While on the ward she was largely ignored by the medical and nursing staffs.

Another patient was quiet and did not disturb anyone, but made it plain early in the game that he saw no sense in the therapeutic program and failed to show up for most of his PT and OT sessions. He too was soon discharged.

Another patient who developed a reputation among the nursing staff of being intractable died shortly after her therapy started, and thus we had no chance to see how the pattern would develop over time.

For sustained intransigence we must look outside our sample of sixty. Helga Schmidt was not on rehab while we were there, but hung out in the general rehab area much of the time and was notorious to the veterans on the rehab staff. She carried on a steady campaign of criticism of the hospital, its staff, and associated public agencies, and was constantly demanding attention for her ills and wrongs. She was regarded by most with some amusement as a "character." (Any unit or institution—except the most oppressive—can tolerate a few such characters, and they may make life more interesting by adding a little spice. But if their number goes beyond a few, they become a threat which must be contained.)

Linda Witt continually and bitterly attacked the staff to

anyone who would stop to listen to her. She refused certain
tests and claimed that they made her condition worse. She regarded herself a prisoner who was improperly being held
against her will. She was considered crazy by most of the staff
and transferred off rehab soon after she refused to take some
diagnostic tests.

Samuel James was the most clear-cut rebel of those on rehabilitation for a long period of time. It was not that he refused to cooperate in treatment. In fact, he carried out treatment procedures far more faithfully than most patients and
the therapists credited him as being the one most responsible
for the success in maintaining his high level of physical function and avoiding ulceration of the skin in the paralyzed parts
of his body. But he did not accept the imposition of routines
and procedures and would protest vehemently when he
thought his autonomy was being invaded. He was particularly
disliked by the ward staff, whose authority he openly flouted
time after time, and whom he sometimes outshouted, cursed
at, and threatened with violence. He was kept on rehab because he was young and was making good physical progress,
and thus represented a potential dramatic success from the
viewpoint of the therapy staff. But his behavior kept him from
being discharged for over a year and even when he got out, it
was on terms which he did not like—being placed in a foster
home because the staff thought he could not be trusted on his
own. He sometimes used the rehab philosophy against the
staff. For example, when he was temporarily blocked from
going out on a pass by himself, he pointed out that the staff
claimed that they wanted to develop the patient's initiative,
but would not even let you go out on your own.

Much of the intransigent behavior on the unit came from
the young adults, of whom James was one. The most dependent of them often made use of such behavior as a means of
getting more personal care. Thus, Lee Ashby would lay down
the law to the ward staff and make complaints against them
when they did not give him the care he thought he was en-

titled to. Nursing personnel, on the other hand, were more likely to give in to such threats than they would in the case of an older patient, and also the younger patients were more likely to receive support from the more authoritative physicians when they made complaints about inadequate care. Many of the young adults other than James turned on an angry attack at times, but it was more likely to come at fairly infrequent crises. James, on the other hand, was likely to open such an attack almost any time he was crossed.

HOME

Colonizing may well be the most common adaptation in an institution where almost two-thirds of the admissions stay until they die. If you don't have much choice—and those who are seriously disabled and have no funds or interested family or friends outside the hospital have little choice—you may well be inclined, not only to make the best of what you have, but to insist that it isn't so bad a life after all.

Even though rehab selects the most "active" cases, the majority of these patients are destined to stay at Farewell Hospital and some of them come to realize this while they are still on rehab (in a few cases even before they come to rehab). Some of these patients react by carving out a reasonably satisfactory life from what the hospital has to offer. What they carve out often has little to do with the rehab therapy program.

At least six of our sample of sixty fell clearly into this group. This included one man who had been in the hospital for many years already and to whom the stay on rehab was only a rather confusing interlude in the pattern of life he had already adapted himself to.

Barbara Kahl, age fifty-six, although physically able, decided she had no future on the outside and came to Farewell with the expressed intention of staying. She actively entered the patients' social life, got herself a boy friend, took part in many activities—in short, created a new and surprisingly varied round of life in a short time. It is a patient like this who illustrates Goffman's notion that "the staff itself may become vaguely embarrassed by this use that is being made of the institution, sensing that the benign possibilities of the situation are somehow being misused."*

Some other patients gradually come to realize that they cannot make a satisfactory arrangement for life on the outside and look more and more to see what they can make out of life in the hospital. Some of the most clear-cut cases of this pattern were not in our sample of sixty because they were already on rehab when we came. They are not necessarily severely disabled people, but tend to be those who can get around the hospital and its environs fairly easily. It includes, for example, at least three amputees who can maneuver the wheelchairs with facility. They have an interest in some of the activities available in the hospital (for example, games and patient politics in one case, a romantic affair in another case, hanging out with the boys and shooting the bull in another), and the physical and social competence to pursue such an interest. In fact, the almost completely helpless patient—the one lacking in physical, intellectual, or social skills—cannot develop such an adaptation to the institution simply because he has no resources for building a tolerable existence out of the limited materials offered by the institution. Thus, often the relatively self-sufficient patient who faces an environmentally dreary or problem-studded life outside the institution will be the one who takes the colonization tack.

THE PARTY LINE

Another major adaptation of the rehab population is what Goffman calls conversion to the official view. As we pointed out earlier, however, the official view is not a very consistent

* *Ibid.*, p. 63.

one. Most of the staff members center around one of two orientations—the custodial or the therapeutic. The custodial view is upheld mainly by nursing personnel and to some extent by the resident physicians. The therapeutic view is espoused mainly by the higher-ranking physicians (who see little or nothing of the patients), the therapeutic specialists, and the social workers. (Of course, the actual situation is not quite as "pure" as we make it sound here. One does hear therapeutically-oriented statements and see therapeutically-oriented acts on the part of nurses, and a few of the social work and therapy specialists often seem to act more with a custodial orientation in mind than a therapeutic one). To these two staff orientations there are corresponding patterns of patient reaction.

Custodial. The colonizers have married themselves to the institution and gain their satisfactions out of it, but largely in spite of the actions of the staff rather than because of them. The converts to the custodial view, on the other hand, ally themselves to the custodial forces, often cooperating with them, and try to get other patients to go along with this view.

Our two most clear-cut custodial converts are not part of our sample of sixty because they were on rehab long before we came—in fact, their long stay on rehab is probably due in part to their espousal of the nursing viewpoint. (They are part of the old timers group described in Chapter 3.) Sara Kent and Marian Marsh are both severely disabled middle-aged women. In spite of their need for a great deal of service, they tended to be quite patient and did not make the insistent demands for service that was found among many of the young adults. They treated the younger Negro women who worked as aides (both these patients are Negro) somewhat as daughters—they would listen to their troubles, give advice, exchange small talk on matters of common interest. In turn, they received better-than-average attention from the nursing staff, who not only met their physical wants more readily, but also socialized with them, performed special favors for them, and listened to their opinions about their own care and treatment.

These two patients made efforts to induct other patients into the ways of rehab, not so much in promoting enthusiasm for and cooperation in the therapy program, but in trying to get patients to cooperate in the ward routines and avoid making unnecessary demands. Their theme seemed to be: "Play along with the nurses and doctors, do what they say and don't try to push them around, and you will be better taken care of than if you try to act smart or make trouble. Besides, the staff knows best how to run things and we shouldn't try to tell them." This theme seemed to serve them well, but they were much less successful in getting other patients to go along with it.

The custodial line did not have many followers, even among those resigned to spending their life in the hospital. Criticism of nursing and medical care was frequent and patients did not become enthusiastic supporters of a program which they believed did not give them proper care. None of our sample of sixty developed the pattern of relationships to the nursing staff that Kent and Marsh did. Those who tended in that direction were mainly women (never men) of a domestic work or un-skilled labor background. For these women, the nurse or doc-tor perhaps represents a replacement for the one-time house-wife or boss to whom they were subservient and whose authority they did not challenge. (That is not to say that all patients with a servant background took on a custodial line. One patient who most strenuously resisted the ordering of her life by either ward or therapeutic personnel was a person with a background of domestic work.)

Therapeutic. Conversion to the therapeutic tack finds more adherents, as it should in a program where the staff is de-liberately trying to select patients who fit in well with the therapeutic philosophy and program. The fact that only about ten out of our sample of sixty clearly fit into this pattern (al-though some others lean strongly this way) is simply evidence that the selective procedures are not very efficient, or more likely in this case, that the total body of candidates from which the selection must be made does not contain many with the desired characteristics.

Patients employing this tack agree that application to therapeutic training and exercises are a major reason for being on rehab, that a patient should apply himself diligently to such therapeutic activity so that he may become more independent in function and may be able to return to a more "normal" life. Such patients are described by the staff as "well-motivated" and are—from the viewpoint of the therapeutic staff—good candidates for rehab. By acting on this tack vigorously and consistently, the patient can even overcome the initial disadvantage of a poor reputation in his previous record and become, so to speak, a self-made success.

These patients may show definite improvement in physical function and a greater than average proportion of them leave the hospital, usually directly from rehab. But following this tack does not necessarily lead to success. Obviously, a patient with a progressive deteriorating disease may die in a short time despite all efforts on his part and that of the staff to arrest or reverse the pathological process. Others may be in a condition where their useful functioning cannot be improved significantly. In the case of such failure, the patient is likely to be more bitter about the failure than in a case of a patient who had not originally committed himself so wholeheartedly to recovery, or at least to substantial improvement.

The frustration of such a patient is extreme when the therapeutic staff does not respond to his clearly pronounced adherence to their philosophy and his desire to participate in their program. This happens in cases where the patient is so severely handicapped and has such a hopeless prognosis from the viewpoint of the staff that the time and effort spent with him seem wasted. The patient uses the therapy staff philosophy as evidence that he needs and deserves more and better treatment, and when this is not forthcoming, he feels that he has been abandoned by the very people he allied himself to and whose pronouncements he supported.

In some cases the "motivated" behavior of a patient may mislead the staff. So convinced are many staff members that motivation is an essential part of success in rehabilitation, that they come to expect great things from those patients who speak and act according to the therapeutic viewpoint. In some cases, however, the patient's physical condition apparently makes it impossible for him to realize his own or the staff's therapeutic goals. Then, not only is the patient disappointed about his progress (even though he may have made substantial progress), but the staff finds that they have gone out on a limb in building a program on unrealizable goals and perhaps even making promises to the patient which they are not able to fulfill.

Hilda Goethe was one of the rare patients who was able to espouse the therapeutic line and work hard at her therapy tasks and at the same time cooperate with the ward nurses, fit smoothly into the ward routine, and advise other patients on how to get along on the ward without causing any trouble. The fact that these two tacks are seldom combined suggests that they are in part incompatible from the viewpoint of the individual patient. The characteristics making up the best custodially-oriented patients are compliance, passive adjustment to the status quo, and acknowledgment of the authority of the ward staff. From the viewpoint of the therapy staff, these same characteristics are associated with "lack of initiative"—the initiative needed to work hard to improve oneself in therapy, on the ward, and elsewhere.

Patients with a therapeutic orientation are more demanding of therapy and services and are likely to become the bane of the nursing and medical resident staffs. When they believe that they need something—for example, a program of standing or ambulation exercises on the ward—they are likely to demand it, to argue that the ward staff is not doing its job if they do not get it, and to complain to higher authorities about improper treatment. To nursing personnel who do not consider many of these therapeutic tasks as their job, such patients may become a nuisance. Someone like Gloria Crane who not only campaigns for her own "rights" and services, but advises other patients on how to battle for their rights, can be quite upsetting to the operation of a ward.

Relationship of inmate tacks to patient interaction patterns

Patient interaction patterns have been discussed in detail in Chapter 3. The intransigent tack is most closely associated with the young adult group, although except for James, it is not very common even there. Lee Ashby and Lloyd Priest have a reputation for vigorously demanding nursing care and other treatment for themselves. Others have more frequent outbursts than one finds in the rest of the inmate population. The staff consider the group an especially difficult one to deal with. However, the staff do not solve their problem as they do with some of the older patients by simply getting rid of them, because they regard these younger people as more worth saving and therefore are willing to put up with more trouble from them. The patients in this group often make effective use of the therapeutic line to make demands even though their general pattern of behavior does not fall into what we have described above as the therapeutic orientation.

The alcoholics might be expected to be among the intransigents, and they were sometimes noted to be uncooperative in ward and therapy procedures and to become abusive toward staff members. But they did not demand more therapy or better care as the young adults often did. Their complaints and abusiveness were, so to speak, "not part of the program," but were the kind of behavior which they probably would have carried on in other settings as well.

The withdrawal pattern was, as noted before, practiced by the isolates. It was a form of getting away from the ward, from interaction with others, from observations by the staff.

They might leave the rehab unit entirely or stay in their cubicle or sit in the corridor or park off by themselves in the day room. But whatever means they used, they succeeded in largely cutting themselves off from their fellows and staff.

The colonization pattern was found most strikingly among the Jewish group. These were all patients with fairly serious disabilities, but still able to operate independently (except Stephen Pepas after his condition deteriorated and he finally died of his disease). They saw no hope of getting out of the hospital, but they had in a rather high degree the social skills and the hobby and game interests with which to build an active life within the hospital. Their religion and their colonizing pattern were probably an accidental relationship and certainly do not mean that all or even most of the Jews coming onto rehab may be expected to develop this pattern of adaptation. In fact, those who definitely expect to return to the community and whose program is reasonably successful in improving their function do not develop intimate relationships with members of this group simply because they find the pattern of life that these colonizers have fallen into rather distasteful.

The colonizers represent a scattering of patients from other groups and non-group members. The Italian group lean strongly in this direction. One of the respectable women, Barbara Kahl, is a clear-cut colonizer. The colonizers are mostly people with fairly good resources for developing social relationships and other interests in the hospital.

The custodial tack is closely associated with the old timers. They have a good relationship with many of the nurses and nurses' aides and encourage other patients to cooperate with the nursing personnel and the ward procedures. Some of the members of the domestic group also tend in this direction, but none have worked out the smooth modus vivendi that the old timers have. Perhaps some of them will if they are there long enough. On the whole, however, they are more passive in their adaptation and do not try to direct other patients along the same path.

The respectable women are on the whole quite strongly oriented along the therapeutic tack and are rather scornful of their associate Kahl for having abandoned this orientation. Two of the non-group leaders are very strongly therapeutically oriented and even try to sell this orientation to other patients.

We find the therapeutic orientation among a scattering of people from splinter groups and non-group members. There are even a few of the near-isolates whose interaction has been greatly reduced by their very severe disability and who at some point strongly espoused the therapeutic philosophy, but usually became quite discouraged with their lack of progress.

We can also spot a few "burned-out therapeutic converts"—patients who started with a strong acceptance of the therapeutic rehabilitation philosophy and became embittered with their lack of progress. Such a person can easily become a subversive critic of the program, seeking adherents to such a destructive line among other patients. We found very few on rehab at any given time, probably because such patients are discharged rather quickly when they reach the point where they are vigorously criticizing and subverting the program.

Playing it cool

Most patients do not stick closely to any of these tacks, although they may lean more strongly toward one than toward another. Rather, they "play it cool." "This involves a somewhat opportunistic combination of secondary adjustments, conversion, colonization, and loyalty to the inmate group, so that the inmate will have a maximum chance, in the particular circumstances, of eventually getting out physically and psychologically undamaged."* Their pattern of adjustment may also be altered through time.

An extreme type is the "sharp operator," who quickly dopes out the biases of the people he has to deal with, espouses their

* *Ibid.*, pp. 64–65.

line when in their presence, gives only as much information and control over himself as is consistent with getting a particular therapeutic job done, and provides for his own needs as much as possible. This style of adjustment requires a considerable amount of independence in physical function, intelligence, and self-confidence in dealing with people in a more authoritative position. These requirements eliminate the great majority of patients. A good example of this style is Gaston Ugeny, who told enough about his background to indicate that he had some college education and was employed in a semiprofessional job, but always managed to dodge inquiries about his finances. He was able to get conditioning exercises and treatment for infected skin ulcers but refused to commit himself to a long-term follow-up program. On the ward he took care of himself in large part and thus avoided demands on the nursing staff. When the time came for discharge, he arranged this himself. Some of the staff, especially the social workers, were annoyed by his reluctance to discuss some aspects of his life and his activities, but at the same time they admired his self-reliance and had so much confidence in him that they were quite willing to let him make his own discharge plans and launch himself back into the community on his own— something they do not usually allow a patient in his physical condition to do.

Other patients, though not as adept as Ugeny, sometimes managed to get what they wanted from rehab without accepting any part of the rehab pronouncements. Thus, John Young wanted simply to get a prosthetic leg and training in its use. The rest of the program he ignored and sat out his time until he was walking on a prosthetic leg and ready to go.

An intransigent stance, an open verbal attack upon the staff or the program, is usually brief—the product of someone "blowing his top." But sometimes such an attack can be used in an opportunistic manner as part of the game in promoting a successful career on rehab, as in the following material from our field notes.

Tudor was a patient who had been around rehab for a number of months and was listed for today's team meeting as a discharge case. There was a brief discussion of his case and then he was brought in in a wheelchair. He promptly backed his wheelchair up against the wall as far away from the semicircle of staff as he could get. Faber (physical therapist) had already reported that Tudor had complained about pains in his stomach during some of the exercises. Faber said he had been taking it easy on him for that reason. Ramirez (resident physician) questioned Tudor about whether he felt any pains and Tudor talked about some pains in his leg and in his stump on his amputated side, but did not mention his stomach. Ramirez repeated the question in slightly different form several times, but got no information about his stomach pain. When Ramirez appeared through with his questioning, Berger (attending physician) remarked to Tudor that that was all they needed him for and they would see him at 1:00 this afternoon in the PT gym for a further discussion of his case. This was the remark that started Tudor's outburst. It went along the lines of: "Discussion, discussion, that's all you people think of, discussion. Month after month I hear nothing but discussion, but I never get out of this damn place." He went on for another minute or two while Faber was standing there holding the door open (and thus the patients outside the room could hear this tirade also) while Tudor told about the sick wife he had at home whom he wanted to take care of, about the fact that there was absolutely no necessity for him to stay here any longer, that if they were going to do something for him, they had plenty of time to do it already and they had just been fooling around all these months, that he was thoroughly sick and tired of all this discussion with no action ever being taken and if they didn't get him out of here today, he was walking out anyway. Several times, he hurled challenging questions at the physicians such as "If you were going to do something about my leg, why didn't you work on it a long time ago?" After each such question, he would pause as if waiting for a reply. He was met with complete silence. His whole outburst did not get a single response from any of the physicians or other staff members, all of whom just sat there stonily staring back at him.

Tudor's outburst, although it got no response during the meeting, got rather quick results after it. That afternoon he was placed first in line among the group of amputees whose cases were being reviewed. Two days later he was discharged to his home, a process which would have taken at least one week and more likely two or three weeks if he had not applied this angry pressure. It was fairly clear that much of his anger had been "put on." He was chuckling later in the day about the way he had made the staff sit up and take notice and got them to work on his case more rapidly. He did not appear in later conversations to be nearly as anxious about the sick wife as he had been during his morning public tirade. However, he did think that the staff had been dragging their feet on getting him out of the place and a little jolt of this sort would speed things up.

Such attacks do not often occur even among those who are bitterly critical of some aspect of the hospital, the program, or the staff, or who believe that their case has been thoroughly mishandled. Most of the inmates have social backgrounds which are conducive to their making a docile presentation to authority. The previous social status of most was low and their associations outside of their families and neighborhood clique were usually with their "betters," to whom they were expected to show deference. The vast majority are now receiving aid from the department of welfare and many of them were receiving such aid even before they were institutionalized. Welfare has access to the most detailed information about them and their relationships and can coerce obedience in some important respects. Most have been in institutions for several months or years—institutions which are designed to work smoothly with unthinking compliance from the inmates and get thrown out of kilter by questions, demands, and complaints. The rehab unit is part of such a great compliance-demanding organization. True, one finds on this unit some staff members who are interested in promoting individual initiative on the part of the patients, but the area for such initiative is severely restricted and it is obvious even to the relatively uneducated and unintelligent patient that individual staff members are not free to expand these boundaries appreciably.

There is a pervasive fear among the bulk of the patients of getting into trouble, of getting a bad reputation among the staff. Even some of the more self-directed and therapeutically-active patients agree that lack of cooperation "doesn't pay." When some of them can be pinned down to just what they are afraid of, they give replies such as the following.

Some amputees will maintain that if you complain about the long time it takes to get a prosthetic leg, about getting it properly adjusted, or about getting discharged afterward, staff members, department of welfare authorities, and prosthetic dealer representatives will punish you by making you wait even longer. Some patients suggest that complaints about nursing care will be met with the withdrawal of goods and services by ward personnel. "If you make trouble, you'll end up by not getting your pajamas or any soap or any toilet articles." Some say that if you prove troublesome to the staff or talk back or make complaints about them, you will be thrown off the ward, and they will often cite cases of a patient who is discharged a day or two after he was overheard making an angry complaint about some aspect of the rehab service. Since most patients regard the rehab unit as a more tolerable place to stay than other units in the hospital, a belief that they will be punished in this way can be a strong sanction.

In short, many of the patients see the staff—especially the nursing and medical resident staff—as a rather powerful force which can and sometimes does punish trouble-makers and complainers. These patients believe that you at least have to make a show of cooperation with the staff if you want to stay on the unit and receive the care that you believe you require. Some patients, too, are concerned about simply maintaining a reasonably friendly relationship with ward staff and they believe that if they "get nasty" with staff members, the staff will end up no longer talking with them or listening to any further complaints. Some of the more dependent patients who need constant care are afraid that this care will become worse as their reputation with the staff deteriorates and that they might suffer physically as a result. John Green, a severely disabled paraplegic, maintains that he is often not helped out of bed or into bed at the proper times, that his skin is not taken care of thoroughly enough and often enough, that the dressings on his infected areas are not changed when they should be. He points to one of his fellows, Lee Ashby, as a man who gets much better care from the nursing staff as a result of frequent angry outbursts, threats made against the nurses and aides, and complaints launched against them to higher authorities when he thinks they are not doing their job right. Green, however, says that he tries to contain his anger against the nursing staff because they would not like him and perhaps would not even talk to him any more if he acted the way Ashby does, and that his complaints on other matters would also be ignored as additional punishment. (The fact is, however, that although Green keeps himself in check most of the time, he has uncontrollable outbursts now and then and as a result has a bad reputation with the nursing staff, anyway. However, his complaints have not been consistent enough or well enough directed to really make any difference in the kind of care he gets. Thus, he has succeeded in getting the worst of both possible worlds.)

Even the demonstration of a patient surviving a bad reputation and getting better care does not seem to reverse the more common pattern of compliance and docility. Thus, though Green maintains Ashby gets better care because he makes his anger known, Green does not want to take this path himself. Even though Gordon Newell describes an incident in which Samuel James cowed the kitchen and nursing staffs into giving him more food when they did not want to, Newell says he would never do anything like this himself and he believes most of the other patients would not because "they're scared."

However, if uncooperativeness doesn't pay, neither does docility. Thus, Samuel Nash went through periods when he tried exercising patience while waiting for something to be done for him or some information to be brought to him. He would simply sit back and wait to hear about what was happening to the electric wheelchair which had been removed suddenly for repairs. He would wait patiently to hear more about the transfer he had requested which a physician had tentatively agreed to. He went through a period of waiting patiently for a physician to order a new battery for his wheelchair to replace the one that had gone dead. Each time that he would try the patient waiting technique, he would simply be left waiting week after week until he finally reached a point where he made an angry demand about the matter, after which he usually received fairly prompt action. The experience of other patients too was that waiting usually led to being ignored. The long periods of time which so many patients spend on rehab is in itself an illustration of the fact that with a largely docile population nobody need rush to get things done. If it is true that angry outbursts, complaints, and demands for action turn staff members against patients (as many patients maintain), the patient may simply have to make a choice between being liked and getting service.

Living in the cracks 8

"Without something to belong to, we have no stable self, and yet total commitment and attachment to any social unit implies a kind of selflessness. Our sense of being a person can come from being drawn into a wider social unit; our sense of selfhood can arise through the little ways in which we resist the pull. Our status is backed by the solid buildings of the world, while our sense of personal identity often resides in the cracks."*

*Erving Goffman, *Asylums* (Garden City, N.Y.: Doubleday, 1961), p. 320. A detailed exposition of secondary adjustments with illustrations from a variety of total institutions is found on pp. 188–320. Readers of

Even where we have the best-intentioned, hard-working, dedicated caretakers and therapists, the inmate will not have all his needs fulfilled by the program in the way he wants. The facilities and the staff work schedules are simply not structured to take all the inmate's desires into account. In fact, in some instances they will be an obstacle to the inmate's securing his wants. This is true of all situations where individuals become a part of an organized structure. (It is just as true of staff wants, of course, but we will consider here only the effect on the inmates.)

Much of the life of the Farewell Hospital patients, including those on rehab, must be "in the cracks." Such "secondary adjustments" must serve them whenever the standard official path does not lead to the goal they consider desirable—or else the goal must be changed. The therapeutic converts can perhaps most readily live according to formal organizational procedures and goals, but even they often find that things do not go the way they are "supposed to" and that even the active therapeutic life must be improvised to some degree. Besides, the therapeutic staff's philosophy comprehends only a portion of the issues that the inmate must face—the rest of the issues require some kind of treatment outside of this philosophy. Patients without the therapeutic tack must pursue an even greater proportion of their goals through secondary adjustments. We intend here to give some illustrations of how such adjustments serve the patient on the rehab unit.

Making do

What do patients do when they believe they are not getting proper care through the prescribed route? One way to get things done is to do them yourself. For most of the more physically independent patients, this is the preferred path.

Goffman's essay will recognize our debt to his conceptions, including much of the terminology used in this chapter.

Almost all do their own eating, dressing, and washing, even though some aspects of these activities may be difficult for them. For example, a few men cut themselves quite often when shaving, but they usually prefer to try it themselves rather than to ask to have it done for them. Most patients try to get around by themselves in wheelchairs, no matter how clumsily and how slowly they do this. Patients frequently make their own way to the PT gyms by wheelchair or on foot even though they have been placed on the messenger service (the latter implying that the physicians do not think they are in a fit condition to come on their own). The most successful paraplegic patient made a point of keeping the lower part of his body in frequent motion and provided much of his own skin care to prevent the development of skin lesions which were so common among his fellows. Some patients who feel they are not being given enough exercise in the formal program will do some on their own. When a patient's visitors put her through some exercises, it aroused considerable interest among a number of other patients, who proceeded to imitate what they observed. Some patients will work on trying to provide their own discharge if they believe that the social workers and department of welfare agents are not working hard enough on their cases. A few patients succeeded in obtaining hobby materials from the outside when the materials they got from the occupational therapy department proved unsatisfactory or insufficient, or when they objected to the policy of the OT department that two out of every three of the products (e.g., wallets) be contributed for sale by occupational therapy to support the purchase of more supplies.

Patients who are quite severely disabled will sometimes go to considerable lengths to avoid having to depend on the ward staff. At one point Cyrus Brock managed to get back into bed by himself from his wheelchair despite extremely weak extremities. On his own he worked out the procedure of moving his wheelchair close to the head of his bed, slowly

extending one arm along the head of the bed until he was
able to grip the opposite side, turning his body and moving
his head and chest across part of the bed until he could get
a grip with the opposite arm, and then slowly dragging himself into bed. It was a drawn-out, difficult procedure indeed,
and Brock was observed taking about ten minutes to get into
bed by this method. When asked why he went to all this
trouble rather than wait for the ward staff to put him back
into bed, he replied that he often had to ask many times and
wait a long time to get anyone to put him back and that a
few times when he had requested being put to bed, an aide
had spoken to him in an ill-tempered manner. In an effort to
avoid rebukes and long periods of waiting, he had worked
out this method of getting into bed on his own. Brock, however, continued to deteriorate and eventually was unable to
get himself back into bed even by this very slow and difficult
method. Once again, he was thrown back to dependence on
the staff whom he did not regard as dependable or friendly.

Just getting to see certain people in an effort to get information, make a request, or enter a complaint is often difficult.
Some patients can be found lying in wait for physicians, social
workers, and others whom they have not been able to see even
after making several requests through the formal channels.
Patients may wait for the people they want to see at strategic
spots. Parking along the "passageway" in the day room is a
good way to catch resident physicians and social workers who
usually come through this way to see patients or to check
patients' charts or talk to nurses. Sometimes these people
will not stop even if called to, but there is always a good
chance that a sufficiently aggressive approach will cause them
to pause and give the patient a chance to make his wants
known. Those who are sufficiently mobile may pursue these
people in corridors and perhaps to their offices if they know
where they are. Some of this is done quite actively, patients
roaming through the corridors until they spot the person they
want to see and then stopping him in the hall or perhaps

going directly to his office. Some of them try to be a little more subtle, placing themselves in a position where the person whose attention they desire is sure to see them and hoping that this will remind him of something he has promised to do but has apparently forgotten. Thus, Nash parked himself in his wheelchair in the hallway outside of the classroom where the prosthetic clinic was being held with the hope that the physician in charge, upon seeing him there, would remember that he was supposed to order a battery for his electric wheelchair.

Patients work on their own, not only to fulfill their physical needs and to effect discharge from the hospital, but also to promote their social life. Some of them do not want to be dependent on staff-supervised programs for their social activities and try to develop some on their own. They may be successful in getting equipment for hobbies and pastimes. They can move around the hospital seeking the society of more congenial patients. They sometimes start games on their own.

The more dependent patients have the most difficult time and usually make the most bitter complaints about their care and treatment. They are the ones who are unable to do many things for themselves. For them the hospital life is a constant struggle to get help. They find that they are often not transported to an examination, treatment, or social area even when it has been scheduled in advance. They are often not given the prescribed medicines, dressings, or other materials. They are frequently not turned in bed when they are supposed to be. They may be got up out of bed too early or too late, and left sitting up for too long a time until the position becomes extremely uncomfortable and even painful. They are often not fed until the food has turned cold.

They find that their simple daily needs require careful planning. Thus, if you need a bedpan, you have to try to figure out when an aide is most likely to be available. You not only have to get the aide to bring you the bedpan, but if you don't want to be left sitting on it for an uncomfortably long time, you also must calculate whether the aide is likely to be available again in another fifteen or twenty minutes. Thus, such a patient must take into consideration the aides' meal hours or the time that the aides are busy with certain routines elsewhere and must make allowances for this if he wants to get the service that he requires at the appropriate time. On the active rehab unit there are no signal cords for patients, and shouting is usually ignored.

The patient must think carefully about asking to be taken out of bed because he may not be able to get anyone to put him back until he has been up so long that his position has become extremely painful. Such a patient must plot out a radio schedule well in advance and select a station where most of the desired programs are, because once he has managed to get someone to tune it in, he may not be able to get anyone to change it to another station for many hours. When he is finally face to face with the physician, nurse, social worker, or other person he has been trying to see, he had better be ready with the entire list of issues, demands, and complaints that he has been saving up because he may not get another chance like this for days or weeks. All such planning "takes brains." Thus, the patient who is brain-damaged or otherwise low in intelligence and also physically dependent is in a sorry state indeed, unless he can find some special protector or helper among the staff, among other patients, or among outsiders who come to see him frequently.

Getting help

Help from other patients often proves valuable, especially to the more dependent patient. He will get help with such things as changing a radio station, picking up something he has dropped, plugging in a battery charger for an electric wheelchair, taking a message to the head nurse, buying something at the canteen, making a phone call. A few dependent patients even get themselves pushed around the hospital by fellow patients who are in much better condition. In the case of men and women this becomes a courting pattern with the man pushing the disabled woman's wheelchair. (Of course, this might work in the other direction with a woman pushing around a more disabled man, but we never observed this.) Not only completely dependent patients, but some who are dependent in particular ways may be helped by their fellows. A girl who is in generally good condition, but has virtually no use of her hands, is frequently helped by other patients to smoke cigarettes. One patient who often helps her has almost no use of his legs and she will on occasion move his wheelchair into position for him so that he can, for example, get off the parallel bars (two parallel handrails several feet apart used for support) by himself without having to wait for one of the staff.

There were a number of cases of patients helping to find the means for another patient's discharge. Tom Ormsby, for example, at one point made a number of contacts with the relatives of his fellow patients in an effort to find a room on the outside when the standard procedure through the department of welfare had not produced results for several months.

Mutual help by patients can keep the more dependent patients from having to rely so heavily on the staff, who often do not do what a patient wants, and at the same time this help can serve as a means of developing social interaction among the patients.

One way to get better treatment is to pay for it. This, however, is quite rare because most of the patients on rehab have very little money. Only one of the patients whom we observed closely had generous amounts of spending money and he used this to gain some improvement of his condition. He often had other patients do errands for him, even though he could with some difficulty do most of these things for himself, and he always paid the patient doing the errand by giving him a tip. He stated that he tipped aides to get him a better wheelchair early in his stay and at a later time there was evidence that he continued to tip them to receive better care when he was drunk. He was able to get some special dental care usually not given to patients by paying for some service not provided by the welfare or hospital departments. He often bought food at the canteen when he found the regular meals unsatisfactory. For his own entertainment he bought articles not available to most patients, for example, providing his own TV set right in his cubicle. He supplied himself more generously with reading material than most patients could afford.

Patients sometimes try to get a staff member on their side on a particular issue in an effort to dodge complete reliance on formal channels. Thus a patient may try to get a physician to intervene with the social worker to get a desired placement outside the hospital. On the other hand, he may try to get a social worker to intervene with physicians and nurses to get a change in his treatment program. He may try to get a physical therapist to press for getting him a prosthetic leg when a physician seems reluctant to do so. Several Spanish-speaking patients took advantage of the fact that most of the residents were Spanish-speaking to get a more sympathetic hearing for their wants and their viewpoints than patients usually get.

There is no doubt that patients with effective outside helpers or defenders receive better care and are more likely to be discharged than those without this advantage. The most common outside help comes from members of the family and friends whom they had before being institutionalized. This source of help is certainly not available to all and probably not to the majority of the patients. Of our sample of sixty, twenty-one had no connection with family or friends at the time they came on rehab and another twenty-one had some family or friends who showed a modicum of interest in them but did not aid them in any specific way. The remaining eighteen received help from families or friends in the following ways:

Arrange discharge	11
Pressure staff for improved service	5
Provide the patient with nursing care	5
Get information about case and pass	
it on to patient	8
Do favors on the outside, e.g., buying	
things for patients	10
Provide patient with money	3

The ways in which help was given total more than eighteen because in some cases the patient was helped in more than one way. The numbers here are minimal ones. Patients may have received some help from the outside that we never learned about, so the ones enumerated here include only those on whom we have definite information. The item "provide with money" is particularly likely to be inaccurate because patients were reluctant to talk to anybody about any additional source of income for fear that the money would be confiscated by the welfare department.

Carlos José worked hard at improving his function so that he could learn to shave himself, but until such time as he was able to, he arranged for one of his sons to come in frequently to shave him so that he would not have to ask the nurses to put him on the barber list. Allen Putnam received a substantial part of his nursing care from his wife, who visited him every day, fed him at least one of his meals, frequently washed him and changed some of his clothing, kept his bed sheets straightened, tuned in his radio, and in general made him more comfortable. Most of these are things that Putnam would have had considerable difficulty getting done with any frequency by the ward staff. Heinrich Dauterman had much of his grooming taken care of by his sons, who also undertook to transport him to the various therapy areas that he was scheduled to go to. Dauterman therefore did not suffer from lapses in the messenger system that plagued many of the other more dependent patients.

The rehab staff wants patients' families to be interested in their family members who are patients on the unit, but they do not want them to be *so interested* that they interfere with rehab service procedures. They like family members to come to visit and keep patients in good cheer, to provide physicians and social workers with background information, and to provide a place for the patient on the outside when he is ready to leave rehab. However, when the interest of the family members reaches the point where they begin to demand detailed information about the case and perhaps even start snooping through the patient's records on the ward, demand more or special treatment, or raise objections to some aspect of the treatment program or the hospital routine, the family's interest begins to be looked upon as interference. Some of the staff members, especially the physicians, may then feel justified in telling the family members that they are butting into things that are none of their business.

Other outsiders are sometimes helpful to patients. In the case of Jessie Maitland, the members of her church helped her out in a number of ways and her clergyman was particularly useful in acting as a protector against the demands of the hospital and the welfare department. He prevented her apartment from being entered for purposes of investigation and possible seizure of property, and also made it possible for her to leave the hospital on short notice when she decided that she was not getting proper treatment on rehab.

An outside private physician with an interest in the case of a patient on rehab can be particularly helpful to that patient in seeing to it that he receives more effective attention. None of the patients observed had such a physician. So far as we know only one of our sample of sixty was admitted directly to rehab from the outside through the intervention of a private physician who wrote to the director of the service, but even this patient did not receive the special attention that he had expected.

Some patients become part of a special protective group. One of our patients was a Greek who found no fellow Greeks on rehab, but found a small group of them in other parts of the hospital. He was soon spending a large part of his time with them. Not only did they share some of the same past experiences as well as the same language, but they also sponsored a series of social gatherings independent of the staff-sponsored programs and thus made themselves to some degree independent of what the hospital had to offer. Such special groups may provide the patient with more help than he could expect from casual associates, as well as getting favors done for him by other patients, by families or outside organizations associated with the special group, which may even be helpful in finding placement outside of the hospital.

Transportation may be a considerable difficulty for the more helpless patient, and in fact some of these patients must resign themselves to being left in one spot for hours at a time and rarely getting off the ward. A few such patients have buddies who spend much time pushing them to various parts of the hospital. A few others have relatives or friends who come frequently and will take them to the canteen or out-of-doors or elsewhere. There are a number of others who make a practice of hitching rides from whoever comes along. They will talk somebody at their place of origin into taking them along when they are going down the hallway, telling this person to leave them off when he turns in a different direction. They will then sit there in their wheelchair waiting for someone else to come along going in the correct direction and ask for an additional push. At elevator points they can get the elevator man to put them on the elevator and take them up and down. By a series of pushes by different people in the same general direction, they reach their destination and later get back in the same manner. They will make use of ambulatory patients, visitors, volunteers, and all varieties of staff to accomplish this purpose.

Sources

Other secondary adjustments can be found in the manner in which patients obtain extra food. Food is of considerable concern to many of the patients, especially the older ones. The hospital provides them with three "square meals" a day, but clearly the kind of food, its preparation, and its variety frequently do not please many of the patients. They then attempt to get additional food or different food from other sources.

The hospital has a canteen which serves small snacks and some patients eat there more or less frequently at lunch or in the late afternoon just before the canteen closes if they anticipate a poor supper. However, the offerings of the canteen are very limited, and besides, patients do not often have the necessary money.

A favorite gimmick is to get little snacks through some part of the recreation program or parties. There was a period when group work held a Thursday evening program every week on the rehab unit and coffee along with something edible like cookies, cakes, or sandwiches was always given to patients after the program was over. A substantial number of patients gathered there primarily to partake of the refreshments and some of them in fact came in near the end simply so that they could eat and drink without having to sit through the rest of the program. This program drew a number of patients from other wards, usually rehab alumni, who again often came mostly to eat and drink. Occasionally, one would see a patient whose timing had been faulty and would find that she (it was usually a woman) was extremely upset at having missed this single cup of coffee and two or three cookies. The lunches of a Jewish organization also attracted a number of people primarily because of the food served.

At mealtimes, those with big appetites would regularly take the food from those who did not want it all. At one time José Barro—who always complained that the portions were too small—was eating three breakfasts, his own and that of two nearby patients who did not like most of the breakfast food. James gave Dauterman his boiled eggs so routinely that soon Dauterman was taking them off James's tray without even asking.

Food from meals, from parties, and from visitors may be cached in the patients' lockers and bedside tables. Nursing personnel are constantly railing against such a practice because it attracts vermin, but it goes on in a big way nevertheless. Patients who find something they like very much at one meal may pocket some of it if it is the kind of food which is not messy and save it in anticipation of being hungry later on.

Cigarettes and some of the fancier toilet articles, such as perfumed soap, are not issued by the hospital and many patients cannot afford to buy them. Again, parties where presents are given away and bingo games with prizes are popular with many patients simply because of the desired goods which they might pick up. Some patients who play bingo a long time before winning a game are extremely annoyed to find that all the cigarettes have already been taken by the earlier prize winners and nothing is left except some useless trinkets. Such a patient may leave the bingo game immediately because he had come just to pick up cigarettes or soap and now finds that he cannot get any. One patient who smoked a great deal received some of the free tobacco ration from several other patients and with it rolled cigarettes using toilet tissue for the paper.

Good clothing is another thing that is in short supply for many patients. There was a period of time when many of them were trying to work the caseworkers for the purchase of some desired pieces of clothing. As soon as one patient managed to do this, a number of others decided they would try it too.

Hospital-issue clothing is regarded by the staff as common property to be thrown into a general laundry heap when dirty and the new issue made from a nondescript collection of clean clothes. However, patients who find some hospital-issue clothing which is a pretty good fit may try various ways of holding on to it, such as having it washed at the patients' laundry rather than at the general hospital laundry so that they can be reasonably sure of getting the same thing back again. The patients' laundry, located on the rehab unit, could be used by the patient for personal laundry. Some nursing personnel encouraged this stratagem to ease the problem of trying to find clothing that fit from the hospital laundry.

Some patients find that occupational therapy will not support their pastimes with supplies and equipment, or that support for such pastimes is dependent on being paid for it by getting two out of every three products made by the patient. Patients who do not want to work under such an arrangement may try getting supplies on their own, as did Bryan Werner, and then operating out of the group work lounge or out of their own cubicle, using their own equipment and supplies which they get from non-hospital sources. Thus, Werner did not have to turn over the wallets that he made to anybody else, but could keep all of them for his own sale or as gifts to friends.

To get most supplies, a patient needs money. The great majority of patients are welfare recipients and their spending money amounts to four dollars a month. A few are able to arrange to work in the sheltered workshop, but there they are limited to earning ten dollars a month. Thus, they cannot buy much at the canteen or through the mail or by giving people money to buy things on the outside. However, some patients get extra money from various sources. If they have a close friend or family connections in the community, there is a good chance that they will be given spending money from

time to time, and a few of them apparently get this quite
regularly. The staff knows relatively little about the extent of
receipts of such spending money, because the patients assume
that the welfare department disapproves of this and therefore
they keep quiet about it. The staff is most likely to find out
about such extra money when there is a substantial theft
which has to be investigated. When one patient complained
about thirty dollars being stolen and another one of something
like three hundred dollars being stolen, the question in each
case was immediately raised, "What was he doing with all
that money to begin with?" Occasionally patients can keep a
sizable amount of money out of the hands of the welfare department by having a friend or family member receive some
compensation, insurance, or other payment at an outside address and cash it for the patient. Checks sent to the patient
in the hospital run the risk of confiscation, particularly if they
come in an envelope bearing the address of some agency or
company which is likely to be making a payment, for example, the Social Security Administration. Therefore, if a patient
wants to make an effort to keep some payment in his own
hands, he has to arrange to have the check sent elsewhere.
Some other sources of income were some more or less shady
rackets, such as the selling of sweepstake tickets, or at one
period (before a raid), carrying on a policy game.

Places

We may also consider the places in which secondary adjustments are carried on.

Patients in some cases are interested in getting away from
association with others or from observation by the staff. We
have described earlier how some of the isolates spent large
parts of their days out-of-doors, some in areas remote from
the hospital. The long corridors of the administrative building
serve as a meeting place for couples in the evening.

Some patients eat in the canteen partly to escape their dietary restrictions. They are not without staff observation here, because the staff uses the same canteen and quite often sees patients on the diabetic diet consuming a lot of starch and sugar, for example. It is interesting, however, that the staff makes no effort to interfere with this, at least not at that point. Other more or less "free areas" are the lounge and the corridors next to the canteen where many of the patients hang out. Here, too, the staff does not interfere with patient activities. For example, sometimes fights develop between patients, and nursing personnel and other staff simply look on and treat it much as they might if they were patrons in a restaurant and were looking out at a sidewalk where a fight between several strangers was occurring. These same nurses no doubt take steps to break up a fight between patients on their ward, but apparently they regard themselves off duty and the lounge and canteen and first-floor corridors out of their territory and therefore do not treat patients in the same way in these areas.

For a few patients from rehab and a greater number from other parts of the hospital, the sewing room served as a place where they could carry on a variety of activities which the rest of the hospital had not provided for. Some women took care of household tasks, as the sewing for which the place had been set up, but also ironing of personal clothing. One patient set up a small radio shop on one side of the room. Others used it to make sandwiches and eat lunch when they did not want the hospital meal. The enthusiasm of some patients for the activities in the room is indicated by the fact that some patients were always lined up by the door in the morning and after lunch waiting for the room to be opened.

The activists among the rehab patients are likely to have more access to staff areas and interaction in staff activities. Thus, in connection with group work programs, there were a few patients who frequently helped to prepare meals and to clean up afterward and thus had a chance to mingle with the group workers and their assistants at times and at places where other patients were excluded. From time to time a patient or two acted as an assistant in the OT shop. Several patients with clerical skills and the right attitude did some part-time work in the administrative offices. They thus had a chance to enjoy more stimulating and higher status associations and perhaps get a look into some of the staff secrets.

Patients also have their private territories. Among the rehab group this is most likely to be the patients' cubicles. One of the objections that some patients have to being transferred to the nursing units where there are no cubicles is that they cannot stake out for themselves a clear-cut private territory in the same way that they can on rehab. Some patients may be found in the same area for a large part of the time day after day. Thus Grant Whitfield and Cyrus Brock for quite some time would flank each side of the bathroom door on the men's ward. Others take up a station, usually off to one side in the day room or in the corridor. One of the most notorious private territories in the hospital is that of Helga Schmidt, who might be seen on the patient's telephone in the central part of the third floor a large part of the day, receiving surprisingly few protests from other patients about her monopolization of the phone.

The stash

A primary facility the patients use for their secondary adjustments is what Goffman calls "the stash." Patients' lockers and bedside tables are used as stationary stashes for food, personal clothing, and other property. An occasional patient with a great deal of clothing or other property may at times invade empty lockers or perhaps induce some other patient who does not have much property to keep some of hers (this usually comes up with women) in unused space. Clothes are sometimes stashed under mattresses. Interestingly enough, the ward nursing staff makes use of many of the same stashes that the patients do. Bed linen and hospital-issue clothing are "stored" by nursing staff in empty lockers and under mattresses as a hedge against the frequently empty linen closets. Thus, the nurses' aides and the patients may run into one another's stashes quite often but, fortunately, they usually do not covet the same set of supplies.

More interesting perhaps is the portable stash. It is not considered safe to leave anything of any value in one's cubicle when one goes somewhere else because theft is quite frequent. Besides, if the patient decides he wants something that he left behind, it may be a long way back to his cubicle and, for many of the more disabled patients, a return trip can be a great chore.

Women frequently carry around with them cloth bags filled with the various things that they believe they may need during their journey away from the cubicle. The letter-writing Schmidt, for example, always has a stack of envelopes, stamps, and letter paper, as well as something to write with, so that she has all the materials at hand for the use of other people, whom she traps into writing her letters for her. Men are much more likely to carry things in their pockets. The very disabled patients, such as the quadriplegics, often sit on their wallet and other valuables and instruct trusted people to remove these and put them back again when necessary.

Success in working the system

Patients vary in their ability to work out effective secondary adjustments. For many such adjustments, it is helpful to be able to speak and preferably to speak fluently. How can you argue with staff or get their attention at appropriate times if you cannot speak effectively? For certain others it is helpful to be able to get around fairly easily on one's own, at least in a wheelchair. How can you track down staff or lay in wait for them if you cannot move about fairly easily? Thus both the aphasics and the physically helpless patients are severely restricted except in what they can accomplish through other agents. Allen Putnam, for example, was an acute observer and was soon well informed about the details of the operation of the rehab ward and the hospital as a whole, but the fact that he was confined to his bed, unable to write and almost unable to see, made it difficult for him to put this knowledge into practice to promote his own cause except for a limited degree of manipulation of the ward personnel in getting his immediate needs taken care of. He had a devoted wife who came to see him every single day and by using her as an extension of himself, he might have been a very effective agent of his own case. Unfortunately for him, his wife was very timid and did not want to make any demands or try any tricks on anyone else in the hospital except under extreme provocation. The result was that Putnam had only very limited success in improving his life situation in the hospital through his own efforts. Helpless patients with no interested family were even worse off.

From the point of view of the inmate we might think of "success" as the degree to which the inmate attains goals of his own choosing rather than the goals set for him by the institution. (Of course, the institution usually sets goals for "him" as a class rather than for him as an individual, which is one of the reasons why the two sets of goals are often in conflict.) Each inmate possesses or lacks certain competences for using or manipulating the physical structure and the human associations in an effort to attain a more comfortable or more autonomous existence in a situation designed to subordinate comfort and autonomy to institutional efficiency. Much of this chapter has been a detailing of the actions of some of the more competent inmates (or their protectors) in their striving to reach their goals. The reader should keep in mind that in Farewell Hospital as a whole, the more competent inmate may well be in the minority in a mass of people so disabled physically, intellectually, and socially that they have little capacity for effective striving in any direction other than that dictated by their immediate caretakers.

There is no systematic effort on the part of the staff to compensate for an inmate's disadvantages, although some staff occasionally "make a project" out of a given individual. For example, there is no special effort to communicate with the aphasics to see whether they have any important needs or complaints that they have not been able to get across to anyone in the ordinary course of events. There is no effort to periodically check with the immobile patient to see whether he wants to be moved somewhere. There is no special effort to overcome ethnic distance or the fear of someone not accustomed to dealing with authority to encourage the expression of complaints or needs and to reduce the expectation of retaliation. And this in an institution which serves as a reservoir for the severely disabled, fearful, threatened, and rejected. What this adds up to for the patients is: The worse shape you are in physically, psychologically, or socially, the less likely you are to be able to survive as an individual personality.

Where do they go   9
from rehab?

According to the ideal of the rehabilitation philosophy, the best placement for a patient when he leaves rehab is his own home and an environment which enables him to live his former life as nearly as possible. If his former life was a particularly depressed one, some improvement upon it may be sought. If he has no home and is able to fend for himself or to get along with minimal assistance, a rooming house, boarding home, or foster-home placement may be selected as the next best possibility.

Place of discharge

Of the fifty-seven patients in our special sample who were discharged during our period of observation, only twenty left the institution. (One of these was returned to Farewell before our observations ceased.) The remaining thirty-seven were transferred to another part of Farewell Hospital. (This proportion is almost identical with the proportion of deaths among the total discharges from Farewell, suggesting that the rehab patient is no more successful in escaping the institution than are patients who do not get on the rehab program.) Of the twenty discharged from the hospital, seventeen went directly to their own home, rooming house, boarding home, or nursing home, and three others were discharged to a private hospital, a relative's home, and a nursing home after spending a short time on another ward.

The rehab staff knows that the majority of patients do not reach the goal of leaving the hospital. However, they do hope that the patients will at least improve sufficiently in self-care functions to enable them to live a more or less independent life in one of the self-care custodial units at Farewell Hospital. But even this limited goal is usually not attained. Of the "final transfers" (we are excluding patients who were transferred temporarily to another ward for some specific medical or surgical treatment and then returned to rehab) from active rehab to some other ward in Farewell Hospital from our special sample, thirty-six patients went to other Farewell wards (a suicide on rehab accounts for the remaining patient of the fifty-seven):

Discharged to a self-care custodial unit (not psychiatric)	10
Discharged to a nursing unit other than the two nursing wards under the control of rehab	19

Discharged to the psychiatric ward   2
Discharged to the rehab nursing units   5

Eight of those who went to the nursing units were considered medical emergencies. Two of these died shortly afterward. The fact that the other six were never returned to rehab suggests that the staff members changed their minds about their being good candidates for the rehabilitation program. Even if these eight are subtracted from the total, the number going to the nursing units is still greater than those going to the self-care units.

The reason for transferring patients to the rehab nursing units is dealt with in more detail subsequently. But in two out of three of the cases of discharge to these units, the patients were still highly dependent and certainly would have gone to some other nursing unit if they had not been selected for the units controlled by rehab. Of those who were originally moved to the psychiatric and non-rehab nursing wards, three were later moved to the rehab nursing units, but all these patients were highly dependent. Another three who had been moved to the psychiatric or nursing units were later moved to self-care units. In two of these cases the improvement was not the result of any specific therapy, but rather the gradual spontaneous improvement in self-care (perhaps with informal training and prodding from nursing personnel).

Our information on fifty-one other patients who were admitted to the rehab unit in the four-month period immediately preceding the time in which we collected our sample of sixty and who were discharged from rehab during our period of observation shows a similar distribution of discharges (again, the proportion who fail to leave the hospital is identical with the proportion of deaths among total discharges):

Discharged to their own home, rooming
   house, foster home, or nursing home   19
Discharged to custodial units
   other than psychiatric   11

Discharged to nursing units other than those controlled by rehab	17
Discharged to the psychiatric unit	1
Discharged to rehab nursing units	2
Discharged to city hospital	1

Pardon

Few patients are pardoned in the sense that they go on their way with no further tie to rehab or Farewell Hospital and with no necessity to report to any part of the public health and welfare agencies associated with this hospital. In fact, there were only two such cases among our special sample of sixty. The following material is from our observational field notes:

Albert Hetherton was completely atypical for the rehab unit in that he had no "social problems." He came from a stable home and was expected by everyone to return to it in a short time. He was able to manage his own affairs and make his own plans and really did not need the help of the rehab personnel except for training in the use of a prosthetic leg. He and his wife earned their own living and were dependent on no public or private organization for aid, even for the payment of the hospital bills. He was one of those rare finds in a public hospital: a truly voluntary patient who is not dumped in the hospital, but comes to it through his own free will in order to obtain specific help which the staff's expert training can provide for him. The staff did provide this training in the use of a prosthesis. The patient thought they did a good job. He also pointed out that he was responsible in part for the rapid progress he made because he worked hard and wanted to get out of the hospital, in contrast to most patients who do not seem to take their therapy program seriously.

The staff's reaction to this was to put themselves out for Hetherton. They scheduled more intensive training and worked harder on him to try to get him out faster, both to save him money, which he was paying out of his own pocket, and also because they thought he was a very good case which they were almost certain to bring to a successful conclusion if they worked at it.

Hetherton was not on rehab very long because he had spent a period waiting at home while his prosthesis was being manufactured. He did not come on rehab until the properly adjusted prosthesis was in hand, and he was ready to start his training in using it.

A lawyer came to Farewell Hospital to have his appendix removed. At least this is the conclusion that one might come to by simply examining the time sequence. Douglas Stentor was a practicing lawyer and his wife a registered nurse. They apparently had a comfortable income. Stentor had a private physician who was treating him for arthritis and who sent him to Farewell because he thought of this as a special center for arthritis treatment. Other physicians do occasionally refer a patient to Farewell Hospital and even more specifically to rehab, but in all of the several other cases we know of, the private physician wrote directly to one of the medical school physicians requesting that his patient be accepted for treatment. Stentor's physician, however, apparently wrote to nobody and simply sent his patient into the hospital through the usual admissions procedures. It was more or less accidental that Stentor was even selected for rehab. The physician who had charge of the selection clinic for that day wondered what this man was doing in Farewell Hospital, and apparently took him on rehab mainly as a way of getting him out of the hospital quickly.

However, before any kind of therapy or even evaluation could get under way, Stentor suffered a severe abdominal attack which was diagnosed as appendicitis and he received an emergency operation. A few days later, while still recuperating from this operation, his wife apparently realized their mistake in coming here and had him removed to a private hospital.

Parole

DEGREE OF CUSTODY

Most patients "discharged to the community" are not released from custody completely. With few exceptions (such as the two cases described), the patient continues to have some tie to the public health and welfare system which may take him back into its institutional confines if he cannot make a go of it outside.

There are several "degrees of custody."* The highest degree of custody is to be kept in Farewell. Most patients are, after all, sent to Farewell for "custodial care." Those who are transferred to a nursing home or an old-age home perhaps continue in just about as great a degree of custody, only in a different place.

The next lesser degree of custody used at Farewell is the foster home. The hospital in effect delegates a major part of its custodial function to the foster family and expects certain controls to be exercised by that family over the patient. The staff continues to see the patient at intervals and may ask the cooperating agencies to have him returned to Farewell if he does not seem to be coping adequately with the foster-home situation.

A still lesser degree of custody is the boarding home. Here the boarding-home proprietor acts as proxy custodian for the hospital staff, and the welfare department (which provides aid in almost all such cases) must be satisfied that the patient is being cared for and can take care of himself in this situation. Frequently the patient is seen at intervals at outpatient clinics where his return to the hospital may be recommended if the boarding home does not seem adequate to his needs. The dissatisfaction of the boarding-home proprietor can also result in the patient's return to the hospital.

One of the rehab attempts at boarding-home placement was that of Gay Broyles, a middle-aged white amputee. The staff had decided that she was not suitable for a prosthetic leg for crutch-walking. She was doomed to getting around in a wheelchair. The search for a boarding home was left entirely to the welfare department. No one from rehab bothered to

---

* The conception of the term was developed by Edwin Chin Shong.

check the placement which was finally offered. When Miss Broyles was delivered to the boarding home by taxi, the proprietor was surprised to find that she was a wheelchair case. Apparently no warning had been given of this fact. An effort was made to accommodate her, but because some of the doorways were too narrow, she repeatedly had to call for help to get to the toilet, the bathtub, and other places. The proprietor decided she could not provide such service and Miss Broyles was returned to Farewell rehab a few days after her abortive discharge. Thereafter, she refused to accept any placement unless it was first investigated by a physical therapist to see whether it would accommodate a wheelchair. After nineteen months on rehab, she was still waiting for a suitable place.

The hotel or rooming house exercises a still lesser degree of custody, but the welfare department must approve both the residence and to some extent the manner in which the patient spends his money. In some cases, the hotel manager or landlord may decide that the patient cannot take proper care of himself and cause his return to the hospital. Again, a number of medical and nursing services may see the patient and also have the power to decide whether or not he is managing adequately on his own.

Leona Barry, though seventy-four years old and recuperated from a severe leg fracture, was considered a good risk for a rooming-house placement because of her stalwart air of independence and insistence that she could look after her own affairs. She was placed in a room in a seedy hotel district which accommodated many welfare cases. She found it more difficult to care for herself than she had expected. It was particularly hard for her to go out for her meals. She used substantial amounts of money for tips to porters and cab drivers to help her get about and get her errands done. In a week her month's welfare allowance was almost gone, her room and her person were in a state of neglect. The rooming-house operator called the hospital and said she was not fit to stay there. One of the rehab social workers personally conducted her back to Farewell, where she is now regarded as a permanent custodial case.

Even when the patient goes to his own home it may be a form of custody with family members acting as custodians, often under the guidance of the hospital staff. Here again, a patient may be seen at an outpatient clinic, by the home-care service, visiting nurses service, or other agencies which serve a limited custodial function and sometimes, in conjunction with the family, decide to return the patient to the hospital.

In a mental hospital, the staff wants to be fairly sure that the patient will not commit any obviously harmful acts against himself or others before releasing him. In a tuberculosis hospital, the staff wants to be fairly sure that the patient's disease is under control and he is not likely to be a danger to anyone else before discharging him. On a rehab unit, the staff wants to be fairly sure that the patient is able to have his self-care needs satisfied before sending him out—either taking care of them himself or having someone else care for them. The staffs of all these institutions tend to be conservative—when in doubt, hold onto the patient for a longer period. Nothing gets them into more difficulty than taking a chance with a borderline case and failing.

In the case of rehab, the conservative approach also means that when there is doubt about whether a patient can manage under a greater or a lesser degree of custody, the doubt is resolved in the direction of the greater degree. Thus, if there is doubt about whether a patient can get along living by himself in a hotel, the staff is likely to try placement in a boarding home or foster home (or keep him at Farewell, if these are not available). If one type of placement is actually carried out and fails, placement is next made in a situation with a greater degree of custody. If the release of a partially dependent patient to his family is being considered, the staff decides whether the housing facilities are adequate (e.g., will the wheelchair pass through the bathroom door) and whether the family members will be present when needed and able to provide the necessary assistance (e.g., is the elderly wife strong enough to help her husband from bed to wheelchair and back). Again, doubts are likely to be resolved in favor of keeping the patient in the hospital.

If we think of the custodial system as a continuum with Farewell at the high custody end and the family home at the low custody end, we can see one reason why most patients remain at Farewell. The middle range of this continuum is very poorly developed. The urban area provides almost no specially designed residences for those who need limited protection or care, but who are capable of leading some degree of an independent life. Rooms in hotels and rooming houses approved by the department of welfare are so scarce that patients often have to wait months for placement. Boarding homes are even fewer and almost completely unavailable to white patients, as evidenced by the fact that white patients scheduled for boarding-home placement (a rare event in itself) wait months before a possibility is even checked into. Foster-home placement is still a very small-scale experimental program. Nursing homes and old-age homes all have waiting lists and represent little, if any, increase in independent living in any case. Thus, for the majority of patients it is of necessity a choice between Farewell and their own home. If they have no home of their own or if the facilities in their home are inadequate or the family members cannot be present or do not have the ability or inclination to provide care, the patients who are not ambulatory and independent in self-care, speech, and mental function must stay at Farewell. A development of this middle range of custodial placement would give the staff (and the patients!) a wider range of choice in their efforts to find the most suitable living arrangements within the limitations of the patients' physical function.

CONTROL OF TIME AND
PLACE OF DISCHARGE

In most cases, when a patient is discharged to the community, the rehab staff has very little control over just when and where he will be discharged. The patients, too—unless they return to their own homes and make arrangements with their families, relatives, or friends—have little control over their discharge, are not consulted about the accommodations arranged for them, and are given little warning about the impending move. It is as if a giant hand beyond the influence of both patients and staff were manipulating the discharge game.

Patients are always told in advance that plans are being made to discharge them from the hospital and that an application to find a nursing home, boarding home, rooming house, or hotel have been made. But they usually have no control over, or even knowledge about, the placement-finding procedure. One day the social worker is notified that a place has been found by the department of welfare and will be held for this patient for a few days. The patient must have an answer in a day or two because the place will not be held longer. The patient is presented with a choice of accepting or refusing this placement, knowing only the address, which is usually in an area with which he is not familiar. Yes or no? If yes, the patient has to be ready to leave the very next day.

Sally Perkins, for example, was told on a Friday that a place was available and, when she accepted it, she was told that she would have to be ready to leave on Monday. She knew only the address. She had never been in the area of the city where the place was located. She had not seen the room and was given no idea of what it was like. She did not know whether transportation had been arranged for her or whether she somehow had to manage to get there by herself.

Gay Broyles was told the day before she left that a board-ing-home placement had been found for her. She had not seen it. The place had not been checked by the physical thera-pist to see whether it was adequate for her physical needs. She knew nothing about the area in which it was located. She felt she had no choice, was sent to the place, and found it com-pletely unsuitable for a wheelchair patient. In one week, she was back on rehab and had to take up the long vigil of wait-ing for another placement to be tried. The experience made her more wary, so that when she was offered other places, she was more insistent upon seeing them first and collecting other information than she was the first time.

Among our sample of sixty, there were twenty-one place-ments in the community during our period of observation. (Only nineteen were actually discharged and stayed out of Farewell Hospital during our observation period. One re-turned a week after discharge and is not included in the nine-teen patients discharged, but is included in the twenty-one discharges. One was discharged twice, the first time unsuc-cessfully, thus adding another discharge.) Ten of these place-ments were in the home of the patient or with a relative who took him in. In all of these cases, the arrangements were made by the patient or by his immediate family, other rela-tives, or friends. Two of the placements were in nursing homes—one of them arranged by the family, one of them ar-ranged by a social worker who took a special interest in a given patient and took her on a visit to the home before the final arrangements were made. Five of the placements were in rooming houses or hotels. In one of these cases the patient had friends who helped him find the room and get depart-ment of welfare approval, and he also visited it before ac-cepting it; the other four rooming-house placements were made by the "sudden discharge" procedure. Four placements were in boarding homes. In one of these cases, the patient was taken to visit the home in advance—this was the case of Sally Perkins, who previously had an unsuccessful placement by the sudden-discharge method in a rooming house. The other three who were placed in boarding homes all went out by the usual sudden-discharge method. Thus, we see that it is in the rooming-house and boarding-home placements that the patient is most likely to be faced with having to make a quick decision on the basis of extremely imperfect knowledge unless he happens to have some person on the staff or outside the hospital who takes a special interest in him and assists with the place-finding process.

Some staff members, especially social workers, would like to prepare the patient for the move he will make to a community setting. Their efforts are blocked, however, by the fact that the rehab staff has little control over the timing and the conditions of discharge in the great majority of cases. If the patient is not going to his own home (and sometimes even then), the matter is almost always handled through the welfare department. The housing must be approved by welfare, and it is usually this department which finds the housing for the patient. Most commonly, after the staff has made a decision that the patient should be placed in a rooming house, boarding home, or nursing home, the social worker who has the patient's case will apply to the department of welfare for the appropriate type of housing. Usually, then, the people in the hospital sit back and wait, although we have limited evidence that a knowledgeable "agitator" on the social-work staff can sometimes speed up placement. The patient's preference for location or for specific aspects of the room are usually ignored. The department of welfare eventually offers what happens to be available in the specified category. Some categories are scarce—e.g., boarding-home placement for white patients—and these may take many months. When a placement is finally offered, the patient is expected to make a quick decision on the basis of almost no information. Unless the social worker takes a particular interest in a given patient and is willing to spend much time on the case, he will not get a chance to see the room before making a decision.

If the patient is reluctant to accept what is offered, the inefficiency of the place-finding system may be used as a form of blackmail to get him to accept. "If you don't take this place, it might be months before they find another one and it probably won't suit you any better." An occasional patient can get friends to find a place, but it must still be approved by the department of welfare if he is receiving their financial aid,

Life sentence

Among those who stay at Farewell and in most cases will eventually die there, there is also little choice on their part and on the part of the rehab staff about when, where, and how they will be transferred.

Patients are usually transferred off rehab without previous warning. The doctor has requested that the patient be transferred a few days or perhaps several months earlier. The patient may or may not have been told that the transfer is contemplated. If he was told, he was seldom told on what day or where he would be transferred. One day the ward nurse gets a phone call: "Ward —— is ready for Mr. ——. Send him over." The nurse assigns an aide to get Mr. —— and his belongings ready as soon as possible and send him on his way. If a patient has no idea why this is being done or where he is going, he is likely to be quite anxious. If he shares the common poor opinion of the other wards in the hospital, or if he realizes that being moved means that the rehab staff cannot do any more for him, he is likely to be frightened and/or depressed. The fact that patients usually do not protest vigorously is perhaps merely another indication of how accustomed they have become to having other people make their decisions and control their lives. Patients, in fact, have become so accustomed to the "sudden method" of being transferred off the ward that it does not seem to occur to any of them that an error might be made in their own case when they are suddenly moved without previous warning—although errors of this kind do occur now and then and the patient must be moved back again.

Among our sample of sixty patients, thirty-nine received final transfers to some other ward in Farewell Hospital during our period of observation. Of these, nineteen were moved by the sudden method described above. Another ten of them were also not told anything in advance, but they were regarded as medical or psychiatric emergencies for whom advance preparation might not ordinarily be regarded as appropriate. The remaining ten were told in advance about plans for moving them (anywhere from a few days to several months in advance), but they were never told the exact day and usually were not told what ward they were going to—mainly because the rehab personnel did not have this information, as we shall see later. Not counting the emergency cases, therefore, the sudden method of discharge was used in two-thirds of our sample cases who were transferred to another Farewell ward. This is probably not too far from the proportion for the patient group as a whole.

Some staff members believe that patients should be prepared for moves to a new location and, if possible, have some say about such moves. Social workers, particularly, espouse the philosophy of "preparing the patient for discharge." The fact is, however, that the rehabilitation staff has little control over the timing and the conditions of discharge in the great majority of cases.

The physician decides only when the patient is "ready" for transfer and whether he should go to a nursing or a self-care unit. After that, the transfer request is given to a hospital administrative office, which decides where the patient is to be assigned. The rehab staff does not participate in this decision and usually does not concern itself with it. The physician does not know when the patient will be moved. It may be a few days or it may be several months. Often the social worker is not even told about the transfer until after the patient has suddenly been moved. In one case, when the social worker wanted to have a patient moved to a ward where he already had a close friend, the physician replied that they had no control over ward placement.

When a social worker tries to carry out the preparation of a patient well in advance, she may run into opposition from ward nurses or physicians who do not want the patient "stirred up." Some patients strongly resist the idea of being transferred off rehab. If the social worker starts weeks or months in advance discussing the matter of moving to another ward with the patient, such resistance on the part of the patient may simply be prolonged over a period of time and make things uncomfortable for the nurses who must deal with him every day. The nurses, therefore, may have good reason to believe that the more common method of suddenly springing the transfer on the patient is the preferred approach and, in the case of some particularly "difficult" patients, we may even find the social worker agreeing.

Separation from rehab, then, is definitely not a step into something new and stimulating; neither is it a move to the expected inevitable for most patients. Of course, some avoid the shock of movement by going back to their own home or to their friends or relatives. A few long-term patients in the hospital to whom rehabilitation was only a brief and puzzling interlude can settle back into their previous pattern of life. A few other patients somehow succeed in getting the impression that they are being moved off rehab for some special medical treatment and will return after it is over, even though the rehab staff sees the move as getting rid of the patient once and for all. Only very gradually over a period of time may such patients realize that they have been abandoned. (We have little information on this process because—except for one or two patients, we did not follow the patients very long after they had been moved off the rehab unit.) For the rest, the move off the rehab unit means a wrenching away from a somehow familiar, though perhaps unpleasant place, and disposition in an unfamiliar place with unknown expectations. It is especially disheartening for those who have made little or no progress on rehab—as we shall see, this is the majority —since the hope of improvement which they had in the therapy program is taken away and nothing is offered in its place.

An occasional patient is moved to another ward screaming her protest. But perhaps more typical are those like Maria Navarro, who told the following story after she had been transferred to one of the "back wards" of the hospital's nursing unit building.

> I was just getting ready to go to the PT gym one day and that gym lady was there to wheel me down. Just as we were about to go, one of the nurses stopped me and told me that I was to be transferred over here and couldn't go to the gym. I didn't expect to come here. I thought I was going to stay where I was. I could push my wheelchair by myself. I know I was slow, but I could get where I was going and I wasn't no trouble to anybody. I was even getting to learn how to walk again. I was hurt when they moved me over here. I hurt so much I couldn't even cry. All my life has been a waste of time because it led to this.

The patient's choice

Occasional patients who are transferred off rehab may be able to influence their placement. They may put up the kind of resistance that Sheila Rivera did when they tried moving her to the fifth floor of the medical building.

> Do I look like I'm dead? Should I be in a morgue before I die? They moved me off rehab suddenly in the afternoon without giving me any warning. I had never been on M35 before so it came as a shock. You can smell it when you come around the corner. When you see it, it's even worse. There is one patient crossing herself, another staring vacantly, another going "woo woo" like an owl. All the beds are much too high for me. I told the aides not to bother to unpack my things. I was going down to see Dr. Brimstone right away. He's the one who decides

the transfers. I wasn't there for more than ten minutes. I knew how to do this because Annie Broome had done the same thing when she was transferred to M35 and by going to Brimstone got herself transferred. I don't pay $350 [that is, somebody—presumably the department of welfare—is paying that amount to keep her here] to be off in a combination morgue and death house. Brimstone wasn't there, but the secretary wanted to know what I wanted. I told her I had been to M35 and I wouldn't, stay there. Another lady I didn't know said to the secretary that she knew this ward and she didn't blame me. I told the secretary she'd better get Brimstone here right away because I'd been in this hospital for three years and I knew every nook and crevice of it and I wasn't going to spend a night on that ward. If they wanted to keep me there, they would have to find me tonight. I started crying, too, and while I was there blubbering, the secretary had Brimstone paged. When she finally got him on the phone, she explained what had happened. He wanted to have the secretary deal with me. The secretary insisted that he should come because I would go off somewhere tonight instead of going to that ward. When he came, he was pretty impatient, but he was not as gruff as he had been described to me by other patients. He asked me where I wanted to go if not M35 and I told him I wanted to go to R24. He said I couldn't go there. I said I would go to any ward in this building except M35 and M34. He said he would send me back to rehab for a few days until he found another place for me.

About two weeks later Rivera was moved to R24 (one of the two nursing units controlled by the rehabilitation service). Rivera is exceptional in being able to manipulate the system by herself. Some patients may be able to do it to some extent with outside help, as Betty Bitkus did through the agency of her sister and Dauterman through his sons. A few may get the help of an interested staff person who is willing to go to bat for them on certain issues. Very young patients like Johnny Green are likely to get a lot of sympathetic help at certain crucial points and in fact are on rehab largely because of this sympathy. But all of these constitute a small minority. For most patients, their ward placement is beyond their control. This has to be true; otherwise a few relatively desirable locations would soon be filled to capacity and have a waiting list, while others have empty beds. Although a few favored patients can get a special dispensation now and then, the administrative requirements of the institution must in the end take precedence over personal preferences of the inmates.

Most patients realize that when they are transferred to another ward, this means that rehab cannot do anything more for them, and unless they have someone on the outside who is willing to help them get out of the hospital—or, in rare cases, are in good enough shape to go out on their own—they are likely to be stuck in the hospital indefinitely. If a patient does not realize this when he is transferred, some among his fellow patients are likely to apprise him of the depressing facts of life. This realization is likely to be especially disheartening to the dependent, immobile patients (the ones who always go to the hospital nursing wards) who have great difficulty building a viable life as institutional colonists.

Occasional patients make a deliberate choice to live out their lives at Farewell. Barbara Kahl was ambulant and independent, decided she had nothing left to live for on the outside, and deliberately chose to stay at the hospital even though her physical condition was better than many of those who go out to live by themselves. She turned over to the department of welfare all her assets, except her clothing and other immediately personal property, and entered Farewell Hospital committed to staying there. Paul Canty, also in good physical condition, made the same choice, except that he had no assets to give up.

Most patients have no such choice. If they stay, it is because they are physically unable to maintain themselves and have no one who is willing to assume their care. Some patients, when they find that every effort to get out is blocked, may begin to think of themselves as prisoners. They complain about being held against their will. If their complaints become vociferous enough, they may get a letter from the superintendent explaining their rights, as did one eighty-year-old woman we knew. The letter pointed out that she was not being held against her will, that the hospital and welfare authorities had no legal right to hold her there if she did not want to stay, and that she was free to go any time she wanted to.

This woman was unable to walk and could get around in her wheelchair only very slowly and with difficulty. Her small assets had been taken by the department of welfare when she first came there. She was a widow with no relatives or friends interested in her. She had no room or apartment or any place to go to. She did not have enough money for cab fare into the city, much less advance rent for a week or a month. In what way was she "free" to go? It is precisely this kind of freedom which many Farewell patients possess. Unless interested staff members undertake to obtain a special living arrangement for them outside the hospital—e.g., a boarding home or a foster home—such patients are in effect stuck in the hospital and have no choice whatever about the matter—except perhaps suicide. The crucial importance of having protectors and helpers outside the hospital system—interested relatives and friends—is obvious here.

THE FAMILY AS AGENT OR ANTAGONIST

Among our special sample of sixty, the status of a patient's family relationships and his financial status directly affected his discharge possibilities and sometimes his physical progress as well. Thus, a patient may work harder if he sees before him the good possibility of being discharged to his family if he attains a certain degree of independence. Also, therapists sometimes work harder with patients who are expected to go home to their families than they do with patients who they know are destined to be institutionalized.

Changes in the status of family relationships of our sample

of sixty while the patients were on rehab may be summarized as follows:

No change, family remains interested in patient and tries to help him, sometimes gets him out of hospital	21
No change, has family in area, but they show no interest in patient	9
Family loses interest in patient while he is in hospital and "cools him out"	9
No family, family surrogate, or interested friend in the area	21

The importance of having interested family or friends is shown by the discharge records of those in the different categories of family changes.

In the "no change, interested family" category, eleven out of eighteen were discharged from the hospital (three of this group were not counted because two of them were still on rehab and one had died).

Of the "no change, not interested" category, none of six possible ones had left Farewell Hospital (three of this group were not counted because they died in the hospital).

In the category of those who were "cooled out" by family or friends, two out of eight were discharged from the hospital. One of the two who got out was rescued by a niece after her son and daughter-in-law had abandoned her. The other one was placed in a boarding home after efforts to get her back to her original home had failed.

In the "no family" category, seven out of nineteen were discharged from Farewell Hospital (two of this group were not counted because one died and one was still on rehab). These seven included two nursing-home placements. Of the five others, four were amputees who had received a prosthetic leg and were trained how to walk on it. The remaining one was already ambulatory and completely independent and did not need any physical therapy or other therapy and merely had to wait around for placement.

One may say that, with very few exceptions, in order to get out of Farewell Hospital without going to another institution such as a nursing home, a patient must either be in relatively good physical condition and be able to fend for himself or he must have an interested family or friends who are willing to take him in.

It is also clear that Farewell Hospital is used by some families to get rid of family members. A patient's disability is the excuse for getting him into the hospital and then the family members set conditions which keep him from getting back home.

Beth Bryce's discharge was clearly blocked by her son and his wife. Whitfield was put into Farewell Hospital mainly because his wife convinced the home-care program that she could not take care of him at home. Thaddeus Hull's landlady's desire for him to return to her home vanished when she found that he would be confined to a wheelchair and also had a serious cardiac ailment. Marcia Brant's husband and daughter had been putting her into institution after institution (usually mental) and publicly labeled her an alcoholic in an effort to get rid of her.

For a somewhat more subtle cooling out by the family—and by the rehab staff—the case of Cyrus Brock is instructive. Brock had his disability for quite some time and it had been gradually getting worse for several years. His family apparently believed that they could not take care of him and preferred to have him stay at Farewell Hospital. Rather than bluntly tell him so, they pretended that they would take him home again, but they set conditions of physical independence which he could not possibly meet. Part of this was learning to walk upstairs and also being able to take care of himself so that he could be left home alone. It was to accomplish these deeds that Brock thought he had been placed on the rehab program. He therefore worked hard at this program and badgered the doctors to tell him how to become ambulatory and independent in self-care. The doctors also dodged the issue by suggesting to Brock the things he might try to improve his physical function. Brock in turn pestered his physical therapist to help him with these tasks. The therapist had been told by the doctor that this training was useless and that Brock's condition was certain to deteriorate progressively, but she felt that she was not the one to reject Brock's requests and therefore went through the motions of trying to teach him to transfer, walk, and climb stairs. The staff went along with Brock's excuses that his fatigue and weakness were the result of the hot weather. The deception worked so effectively that when Brock was transferred to a nursing unit, he was still able to maintain that this was a temporary transfer and that he would be back on the program when the weather became cooler, even though the staff saw the transfer as final disposition of his case.

Whether a family can or cannot take care of a patient is a relative matter. Whitfield's wife did in fact take care of her husband for a time when his condition was no worse than it was while he was on rehab. There is no doubt that she could do it again if the hospital facility were not so convenient as a means of disposing of him. Stanley Lombardi's parents and their house were at first described by members of the team as most unsuitable for his care and he was expected to stay on rehab for a long time, perhaps indefinitely. Then his parents were forced by court action to make a substantial contribution to his hospital care. Maintaining that they could not afford this payment, they promptly took home the son whom they previously had said they could not cope with at home. According to information we received from another research project,* Lombardi's family is indeed coping with having their son at home—whether better or worse than he was taken care

* The Continuous Care Project headed by Howard Kelman. This project is following a group of patients discharged to the community.

of on rehab is another question. Our point is simply that one cannot make any absolute statements that a family can or cannot make a place for a patient in their home. We must always state the conditions under which this is to occur.

MONEY TALKS

Returning now to the matter of a patient's financial status, we may sum up changes which occurred as follows:

No change, financially poor	39
No change, financially independent (two of these are very questionable)	7
Income or savings markedly reduced by period of hospitalization	14

It is rather surprising that the last category does not have a much larger membership. We might expect that such long-term hospitalization would be a severe financial blow to most people, but this is not the case. The reason is that the great majority of patients were more or less destitute before they even came to rehab, or for that matter, to Farewell Hospital. Many of them had already been on welfare aid before they were institutionalized, and only a very few patients had health insurance. Therefore, this period of hospitalization was merely a perpetuation of the previous pattern of economic existence.

Ten out of thirty-three in the "no change, poor" category (six of these were not counted because four of them died and two are still on rehab) were discharged from Farewell Hospital. Of these, two went to nursing homes. Of the eight returning to the community, three went to rooming houses on department of welfare aid, two went to boarding homes on welfare aid, two returned to former apartments paid for by friends and family and are now living on welfare aid, and one was taken back home by his family under pressure from the department of welfare that they pay part of the hospital care.

All those in the "financially independent" category left Farewell Hospital except Meg Gifford, who died there. Two of these had savings and only a brief interruption of their earnings as a result of their disabilities. The others had family members or friends (a church congregation in one case) who were willing to temporarily support them and return them to the community. Thus, being able to afford living outside the hospital is an important condition to escaping from it. With such financial independence, the patient need not depend upon the institutional personnel to arrange a community placement. Without such financial help, all six of these patients would have had to stay in the hospital for many months, some of them indefinitely.

All those whose savings or income were reduced by their hospitalization suffered a drastic change in their pattern of life, except perhaps Gloria Crane, who held her job and returned to it after a rather short leave of absence. Only four out of the thirteen (one of this group is not counted because he is still on rehab) got out of Farewell Hospital. Crane was one of these. Another was a boarding-home placement. The remaining two returned to their families on department of welfare aid.

Clearly, money helps to get one out of the hospital. The practice of stripping patients of their assets and blocking them from any income except a monthly pittance while they are in the hospital tends to perpetuate their residential and economic dependence.

Success and failure   10

The philosophy and much of the practice of the rehab program imply that certain outcomes are successes and certain
others are failures. In this study we focus on the "working
definitions" of success and failure expressed by the staff actually treating and caring for the patients. In other words, we
are not taking our definitions from formal statements, but are
constructing them from actual practices we observed—what
patients were selected and rejected, what ones received the
most intensive treatment, at what points and for what reasons
were care and treatment expanded or reduced? For example,
the physical therapists indicated that a patient was worth
working with by assigning him to one of the more skilled,

fully certified therapists, or that he was not worth working with by assigning him to one of the "non-professional" therapists. Several of the patients were switched back and forth from one therapist to another as the estimate of their "worth" changed. Occupational therapists could express the same definitions of worth by assignment to functional or diversional therapy; speech therapists, by assignment to individual or group therapy or dropping a person from the program entirely; social workers, by trying hard to work out a community-placement plan or readily resigning themselves to transferring the patient to a Farewell self-care unit. Using these and other more subtle cues, as well as outspoken evaluations at meetings and elsewhere, we could readily determine in most cases when patients were regarded as a success or failure by the staff.

The elements of success

The emphasis in the program is on improvement of physical function, especially that part of physical function which is concerned with a more independent life for the patient. For example, if the patient's disability makes it necessary for him to be fed by someone else, an improvement of function is a change in his condition which enables him to eat by himself. Eating may be further broken down into parts, such as a patient not being able to eat at all, being able to handle his eating except for cutting meat, and being able to do all of this by himself. If a patient's disability makes it necessary for other people to dress him, it is an improvement if he can learn to dress himself at least in part. This again may be broken down into various parts, such as pulling up his pants, tying his shoes, pulling a sweater over his head. The more steps in dressing he can carry out himself, the more independent he is. If a patient's disability makes him dependent on others for washing and grooming, it is a distinct improvement from the viewpoint of the rehab philosophy for him to regain the

ability to wash his face, comb his hair, shave, cut his finger-
nails and toenails, and so on. Here again, a patient may learn
to do some of these things and not others and thus be equally
or less dependent than he was previously. A patient may also
progress from having to be lifted to being able to transfer
himself to his wheelchair, to his bed, and to the toilet.

Progress in locomotion is also seen in a well-defined sequence—from being bedridden to having to be pushed on a
stretcher or wheelchair, to pushing oneself on a stretcher, to
pushing oneself in a wheelchair, to walking with crutches,
to walking with two canes, to walking with one cane, to walking without support but with supervision, to walking without
support or supervision. Each step is seen as a greater degree
of independence in function. In fact, the therapy specialties
have drawn up some elaborate rating scales whereby the various areas of activities of daily living (ADL) for a given patient can be given a numerical score which can be compared
with the score at an earlier or later time and with the scores
of other patients at a given time.

Using such schemes of rating physical function, we can see
that a patient who starts at a lower level and who moves to
a higher one has improved and to that extent is a successful
rehabilitation case. Thus, a patient who started out on rehab
not being able to move a wheelchair and ends up by being
able to push himself around in a wheelchair on his own has
undergone a definite improvement, while a patient who was
already able to push himself around in a wheelchair when he
came on rehab and is still at the same level of locomotion at
the end of the program has not improved himself and in that
sense is a rehab failure.

There is also some concern on rehab about the patient's
social status and activities, although this is almost always secondary to his physical function. The social aspect is focused
mainly upon discharge and the case is considered more successful as a patient gets closer to his pre-institutional style of
life. In practice, style of life is defined almost entirely in terms

of his housing and household. The greatest success is getting
the patient back to his own home with his family. Next in
descending order are getting him into a home with a relative
or friend, into a rooming house or a hotel, into a boarding
home, into a foster home, into a nursing or old-age home.
The lowest level of success is for him to remain within the
hospital system. In the great majority of cases, the latter
means Farewell Hospital and it is better to have him go to a
self-care unit than to a nursing unit (except for nursing units
staffed by rehab personnel in some cases).

Some staff members, especially in casework and group
work, may have other social goals for patients—for example,
bringing an isolate into a position of greater social interaction
with his fellows—but such goals are incidental to the central
foci of the rehab program unless they happen to forward the
major goals just described. If his social work or psychological
counseling causes the patient to work harder in his physical
therapy and improve his self-care, this would be a contribution
to a central goal. If counseling of the patient and his family
causes the family to accept the patient back into the home,
this would also be a contribution to a central goal.

A successful change may be summed up as a change toward
greater independence. The chart shows graphically the rehab
staff's areas of concern with various stages of dependence-
independence through which a patient may move or in which
he may finally become established. The steps in each of the
chart lists are not intended to represent the whole spectrum
of steps at which patients are operationally classified, but are
intended only to suggest the concept of levels of dependence-
independence. Physical therapists may at times use a more
refined series of steps for classifying "mobility," speech therapists use a more refined series of steps for classifying "communication" ability, and so on.*

The aim of rehab therapy and social-work assistance is to

* The chart and the idea of portraying an independence-dependence
continuum were first developed by Edwin Chin Shong.

GOAL STRUCTURE OF REHABILITATION THERAPY

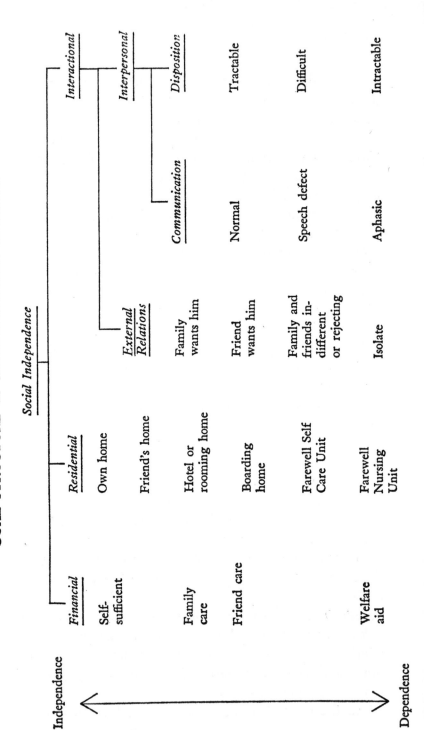

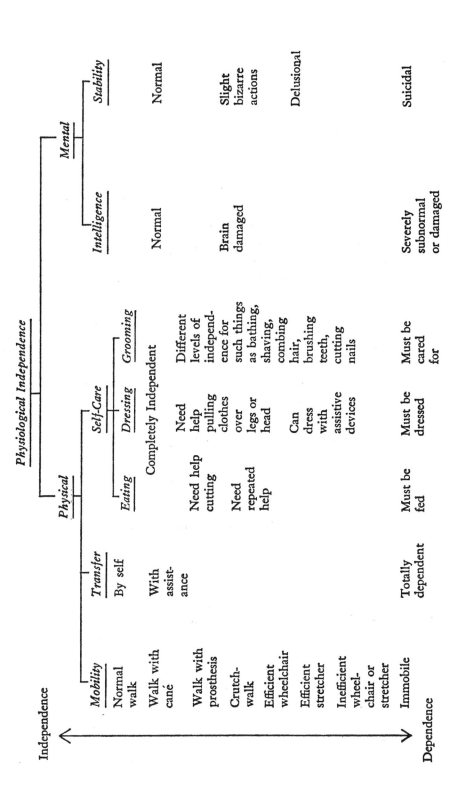

Physiological Independence

Independence → Dependence

	Physical					Mental	
	Mobility	Transfer	Self-Care			Intelligence	Stability
			Eating	Dressing	Grooming		
Independence	Normal walk	By self	Completely Independent			Normal	Normal
	Walk with cane	With assistance					
	Walk with prosthesis		Need help cutting	Need help pulling clothes over legs or head	Different levels of independence for such things as bathing, shaving, combing hair, brushing teeth, cutting nails	Brain damaged	Slight bizarre actions
	Crutch-walk		Need repeated help				
	Efficient wheelchair			Can dress with assistive devices			Delusional
	Efficient stretcher						
	Inefficient wheelchair or stretcher						
Dependence	Immobile	Totally dependent	Must be fed	Must be dressed	Must be cared for	Severely subnormal or damaged	Suicidal

move the patient upward in as many of the areas shown in the chart as possible, although it is recognized that the rehab staff usually have little or no control over some of these areas, for example, the financial area. An upward movement is a success for the given area; a downward movement is a retrogression. The patient who shows promise of making a substantial upward movement in one or more of these areas is a good rehab candidate (but at least one of the areas in which improvement is expected must be physical). If no such upward movement is expected by the staff, the patient is a poor rehab candidate and is likely to be rejected quickly if he happens to get on rehab "by mistake."

How successful?

Using the staff's working definitions of success, we may classify fifty-seven of our special sample of sixty patients into two general groups. The remaining three patients were ambulatory and physically independent and therefore needed no rehabilitation service other than evaluation and placement.

Success (23 cases)

1. Amputees got prosthesis, were
   trained in ambulation, and
   discharged from hospital   5
2. Same as above, except transferred
   to other Farewell ward   1
3. Functional improvement leading
   to greater independence in self-
   care and/or locomotion and
   discharge from hospital*   11
4. Same as above, except transferred
   to other Farewell ward*   5
5. No functional improvement,
   but discharge to home   1

* Of the sixteen patients in categories 3 and 4, eight were independent in self-care at the beginning of their stay on rehab. Two of these patients were in poor physical condition and six of them were in

Non-Success (34 cases)

6. Condition remains the same—
   transferred to self-care unit   8
7. Condition remains the same—
   transferred to nursing unit   13
8. Condition deteriorated—
   transferred to nursing unit,
   psychiatric ward, or other
   public hospital   5
9. Died   5
10. Condition remains the same—
    still on rehab   3

The judgments of success and non-success are based on staff evaluations of the patient's function plus some obvious facts such as whether or not the patient was discharged from the hospital. Success was interpreted liberally. Included as a success case in category 3 was one patient who is still almost completely dependent on the nursing personnel for care. Because the staff—especially physical therapy—considered his condition at discharge slightly improved over his original condition and because his family saved him from permanent disposition in a Farewell nursing unit by moving him to a nursing home (a fate many familiar with nursing homes would hardly consider an improvement), we classify this case as a success. Two other patients in this category were still dependent enough in self-care to warrant discharge to a nursing unit. In category 5 we tabulated a patient who showed no significant improvement in physical function or physical condition during his stay in rehab, but who did leave the hospital to return to his own home even though the circumstances were the rather unpropitious ones of being taken home by his parents after the department of welfare won a court action to force them to pay a portion of the hospital costs. He was

---

good phycical condition. The remaining eight patients showed marked improvement during their stay on rehab and were independent in self-care at the time of their discharge.

thus rated a "social success" for attaining the goal of getting out of the institution. Also included as successes are three people in relatively good physical condition whose physical functioning changed very little while on rehab and who were labeled successful mainly because they succeeded in getting to their own or a relative's home. (All their placements were arranged without the help of the rehab staff; in fact, one of them without the permission of the staff.) These six cases indicate the lower boundaries of the success classification.

The most definite, clear-cut success cases are all those in categories 1 and 2 and the eight with marked improvement in categories 3 and 4. These total fourteen. The remaining nine rated as success cases all showed relatively little improvement and may be thought of as borderline successes.

The thirty-four in the non-success classification had some definite need for rehabilitation therapy, but did not improve in physical function as a result and did not succeed in getting out of the hospital system. They can perhaps be more definitely labeled "rehab failures" in that in terms of the central goals of the rehab program, the patient was no better off as a result of his spending this period of time on the rehab unit.

None of the sixty patients was a dramatic success. Only one-fourth experienced marked improvement in self-care and/or ambulation. A minority managed to arrange discharge from the hospital. There is no evidence of any form of success according to the staff's own definitions in the majority of cases passing through the rehabilitation unit.

Success and time on rehab

Patients who remain on rehab for a short time are more likely to be discharged to a Farewell nursing unit or psychiatric ward. Those who stay longer are more likely to go out into the community, to a self-care unit, or to the nursing unit controlled by rehab (the latter considered by most staff and patients to be more desirable than other hospital units aside from active rehab itself).

The twenty patients from our sample of sixty who spent the shortest time in rehab were discharged to the following locations:

Nursing or psychiatric unit	14
Self-care unit	2
Community (all to own home)	3
Suicide	1

The twenty patients who stayed on rehab longest were discharged to the following locations:

Nursing unit	5
Rehab nursing unit	4
Self-care unit	4
Community (2 to own home, 2 to nursing home, 2 to boarding home, 1 to rooming house)	7

As a check on the consistency of this pattern, we examined an earlier group of fifty-one successive discharges and compared the shortest to the longest third (each seventeen) in terms of length of stay on rehab. The same differences were found in this group.

The short-stay group represents largely a poor-risk population. The first twenty of our sample of sixty includes all but one of those transferred for medical or psychiatric emergencies. It includes four out of the five who died on rehab or shortly after leaving rehab. It includes most of those that the staff consider selection mistakes.

If we use our success ratings, we get the same picture. When we arrange our sample in order of length of stay on rehab, as shown in the table, the sequence begins with eight non-success cases—all about a month or less on rehab. Then there is a scattering of success cases to the midpoint of the total group—all of them more than six months on rehab. In

SUCCESS AND ORDER OF LENGTH OF STAY

Ascending length of time on rehab	Name	Success	Non-Success
1	Powell		N
2	Stentor		N
3	Buber		N
4	Sloane		N
5	Lockwood		N
6	Hollwick		N
7	Adams		N
8	Sklar		N
9	Maitland	S	
10	Breckenridge		N
11	Gifford		N
12	Panaklos		N
13	Bitkus		N
14	Hetherton	S	
15	Heinsius	S	
16	Livingston		N
17	Hull		N
18	Witton	S	
19	DiCresce		N
20	Hart		N
21	Gore		N
22	José	S	
23	Whitfield		N
24	Perkins	S	
25	Kahl		N
26	Gump	S	
27	Pepas		N
28	Keck		N
29	Brock		N
30	Scott		N
31	Crane	S	
32	Young	S	
33	Clemens		N
34	Bryce	S	
35	Barry		N
36	McCormick	S	
37	Goethe	S	
38	Navarro		N
39	Erwin		N
40	Dauterman	S	

Ascending length of time on rehab	Name	Success	Non-Success
41	Sacks	S	
42	Long	S	
43	Lombardi	S	
44	Putnam		N
45	Kraft	S	
46	Bader		N
47	Barro		N
48	Drake	S	
49	Reid	S	
50	Coots	S	
51	Nash		N
52	Adair		N
53	Truman	S	
54	London		N
55	Ormsby	S	
56	Brant	S	
57	Reidy		N

Still on rehab

58	Green		N
59	Broyles		N
60	Adler		N

the first twenty there are four rated a success, only one of the clear-cut variety. The first thirty have seven successes, two of the clear-cut kind. (Of these two, one paid in full for his hospital treatment and had spent the waiting period to get his prosthetic leg at home instead of on rehab as did most amputees; the other had gone through a period of marked spontaneous recovery on another ward before coming to rehab and then paid for his own brace, thus avoiding the lengthy purchase-approval process.) In contrast, the thirty with stays over the median have sixteen successes, including twelve of the more clear-cut cases.

We cannot conclude from this, however, that the longer a patient stays on rehab, the greater are his chances of success.

A certain length of time for treating a given disability comes to be thought of as "normal" and patients who stay much beyond this period usually represent some difficulty of diagnosis, treatment, or placement. Thus, the long-term patients on the ward do not represent clear-cut successes. They are people on whom rehab has not wanted to give up, but for whom little or no improvement has occurred. Among our special sample, those who stay much past a year are more likely to be difficult cases of some kind (usually with placement) rather than the markedly successful. Ormsby was a clear-cut success who stayed well past a year, but the last three or four months were taken up by an exceptionally long wait for a furnished room to be found for him.

The success cases will thus be found mostly among those patients who are promising enough in some way so that they are kept well past an initial trial period, but who do not hang on for many months because of special difficulties of diagnosis, treatment, or placement. This middle group represents the patients who are most attractive to the therapeutic staff because they have the best chance of undergoing a positive change in treatment and do not have the obscure or insurmountable problems which take up so much staff time.

Although the short-stay "rejects" make up a substantial proportion of our sample, at any given time they are a much smaller proportion of the rehab population because they occupy rehab bed space for a very short time. The long-stay difficult cases, on the other hand, make up a small proportion of the total number of admissions or discharges, but a much higher proportion of the rehab population at a given time because they gradually accumulate in numbers.

Roads to success or failure

Locating success and failure among patients is not simply a matter of personality diagnosis or the listing of social characteristics associated with success. Patients are not successful because they have a make-up of "successful traits" or failures because they have a make-up of "unsuccessful traits." Whether or not a given characteristic or action by a patient will lead to success depends in large part on the effect that that characteristic or action has on others around the patient, especially on the staff members and other persons (e.g., department of welfare personnel, family members) who make the decisions concerning the patient's care, treatment, and disposition, and who define what constitutes success and failure. For example, a patient's statements and actions which indicate that he is anxious to improve his physical function and return to the community is not a "successful trait" in itself. Such actions tend to lead to success because the treatment staff respond to such behavior by putting the patient on a therapeutic program, giving more intensive treatment, encouraging him to practice his physical skills on his own, helping him to find suitable placement, and so on. We can conceive of a situation in which the staff reacted to such behavior on the part of the patient by classifying the patient as crazy and referring him to the psychiatrist. In such a situation, the same behavior would tend to lead to failure. In other words, the patient's behavior or characteristics tend to lead to success or failure on rehab according to how this behavior fits into the pattern of acceptable or unacceptable behavior or characteristics in terms of the operational values of those who control decisions made about the patient.*

Furthermore, if behavior leads to success, it does not mean that the staff necessarily likes this behavior. Rather, successful behavior is that which causes the staff to do things which improve the patient's chances of getting the treatment and service he needs to lead to a successful rehabilitation result. Thus, the demanding patient is often disliked by staff members, but

* For an analogous conception of success and failure in academic study, see Julius A. Roth, "The Study of Academic Success and Failure," *Educational Research Bulletin,* vol. 35 (October 10, 1956), pp. 176–182.

his demands may get him the things he needs and thus increase the chances of a successful conclusion.

The way to success or failure is not a neat and automatic
process, with every patient whose characteristics and behavior
are associated with an unsuccessful result soon being eliminated from the program. Reaction to the patient's condition
and behavior varies in effect with the stage of his career, so
that, for example, it is easier for the nursing and medical
resident staff to get rid of an undesirable patient at a very
early stage of his career on rehab than it is at a later stage.
Behavior on the part of the patient which tends to block
proper service from the staff may be more than balanced by
other behavior which tends to encourage such service. Also,
it must be remembered that the rehabilitation program is not
a monolithic one in which there are no deviations from a
party line. There is, in fact, considerable variation and disagreement among individual staff members and various groups
of staff so that a patient who is rejected by one person or
group may well be sponsored by another person or group and
so be able to continue on rehab for a long time and perhaps
to a successful conclusion on the basis of such partial support.

Also, although rehab—like all treatment organizations—has
an ideal of complete knowledge about the patient and a complete pooling of information among staff members so that
the treatment of the patient may be planned and conducted
with all possible information at hand, the fact remains that
such a condition of complete communication among staff
is not even approximately achieved. Important information
available to certain staff members frequently is never com-
municated to other staff members who must make decisions
about the patient. It is not uncommon for a patient to be
almost completely "forgotten" for months at a time if he does
not make a point of calling attention to himself and/or if his
condition is such that no marked changes or "problems" call
the staff's attention to him. Such "communication failures
among staff" and "neglected patients" have often been criti-

cized as deficiencies in a treatment program. Sometimes, however, these apparent defects are advantages from the patient's point of view. It may mean that undesirable characteristics and behavior are overlooked or ignored and the patient is enabled to continue his existence on rehab when a more "efficient" operation would have caused him to be thrown off summarily. During this period of hanging on, the patient's behavior or characteristics may change sufficiently so that when he does come to the attention of the appropriate people, they will consider him a good bet for a further effort.

THE WAYS OF SUCCESS

A patient is more likely to achieve a successful outcome if he is willing and able to act as a coordinator and promoter of his own program of therapy and care. This means he must actively work at getting information about himself from the staff and often pass such information and instructions from one staff member to another rather than relying on communications between staff members to get things done on his own case. He may, for example, pass on to a physical therapist the things which a physician told him about his physical condition which may affect the kind of therapy the PT provides, rather than relying on the PT to learn this from the physician herself. He reminds staff members of commitments they have made to him and demands that these commitments be met. He keeps track of his "official needs," e.g., prescribed medications, being turned in bed, having his bladder irrigated, getting physical therapy on schedule, and he reminds the staff of these needs and insists that they be met. He will apply constant pressure for more care and treatment. He will provide the staff with ideas for his own care and treatment which they may not have thought of. He may obtain or speed up orders for prostheses or appliances through his family or by other means if possible, or arrange repairs and adjustments on an informal basis. He may make an effort to arrange for his own discharge from the hospital. Such efforts at coordination or pushing for more service simply mean that the patient is more likely to bring about these services or actions than if he just sits back and waits for things to be done for or to him and to that extent increases the possibilities of his program being brought to some kind of successful conclusion.

Another type of behavior associated with success is "high motivation," by which the staff means that the patient clearly desires to improve his physical functioning and return to a more "normal" life. This high motivation behavior is often closely linked to the efforts of the patient to coordinate his program, but the two are not the same thing.

The aspect of high motivation behavior which rates highly with the custodial staff is the patient's effort to improve his self-care and to apply this improvement as rapidly as possible in his everyday life on the ward. The nursing personnel encourage this aspect by withdrawing nursing help as soon as the patient shows the least bit of competence in a given area of function. (Although, if help cannot be completely withdrawn, nursing personnel may sometimes discourage independence on the part of the patient by doing something for the patient rather than helping him do it because the former takes less time. For example, it is usually much faster to simply lift the patient from his wheelchair into his bed than to stand by and supervise and help him while he does most of the work of transfer by himself.)

The aspect of "motivated" behavior most visible to the therapeutic staff is the diligence with which the patient works on his therapeutic tasks and his statements that he wants to improve and to get out of the hospital. Such behavior on the part of the patient often causes the therapist to provide a more intensive program and thus makes it more likely that the patient will improve. The therapist encourages the patient to work harder and to raise his sights in striving for improvement in function. The acceptance and open espousal of the active rehab philosophy can sometimes be a crucial factor in whether or not a patient receives therapy. Thus, active therapy was given to Stephen Pepas for "maintenance" even after it was quite certain that he had a progressive irreversible disease, simply because the patient enthusiastically embraced the rehabilitation philosophy and entered all the activities offered to him as far as his physical condition permitted. Herbert Witton, on the other hand, a hemiplegic and aphasic who came on rehab a short time after his CVA (or "stroke") and who was still showing spontaneous improvement during his time in rehab, was abandoned and moved to a nursing unit a few months after his admission to rehab because he made it plain that he did not see any point to the therapy offered to him, often missed therapy sessions, and made a lackadaisical effort in his training when he did come or was brought to therapy. (That Witton was capable of much more physical improvement was shown by the fact that he was transferred from the nursing unit to a self-care unit about half a year later after marked spontaneous improvement of his physical functioning.)

The emphasis on "motivated behavior" sometimes leads the staff to develop unrealistic expectations of the patient's potential. Thus, Joe McCormick was expected to be walking within a short time after beginning his therapy, but was still not ambulating safely when he was released from the hospital after an intensive program of physical therapy seven months later. Hyman Bierman, an eighty-year-old bilateral amputee, had two prosthetic legs ordered for him with the expectation that he would actually learn how to walk on them, largely because he repeatedly stated that he was very anxious to learn how to walk and promised to work hard at it, and because he repeatedly demonstrated both his muscular ability in the upper part of his body and his willingness to exert himself by doing push-ups in a wheelchair at grand rounds (a traditional procedure whereby some patients and their cases are presented to the medical hierarchy for review and discussion), demonstration courses, team meetings, and other places where he could make a favorable impression on influential staff members. In such cases where the staff is misled by the patient's enthusiasm, staff members later suffer disappointment with the results of their program efforts, but still the patient benefits by getting a more intensive program than he would otherwise have received, and by getting appliances, prosthetic devices, and perhaps community placement which the staff otherwise would not have obtained for him.

The desire to return to the community is another factor which increases a patient's chances for success, and in fact such a desire is often linked to what the staff classifies as "high motivation." It is especially likely to elicit increased help from social work. Of course, if no "realistic" plan or effort by the patient or his outside helpers is made, the claim that he wants to return to the community may eventually be dismissed as "just talk." The patient has a big advantage if he has some facilities for getting out. If he must depend entirely on the social workers and the department of welfare, his chances are not good unless he shows marked recovery in physical function or was in quite good physical condition to begin with. The patient with financial ability (which is rare) or with outside help (usually his family) to maintain a place to go to is thus in a favored position. Mary Anne Kraft, Hilda Goethe, and Jessie Maitland were not safe ambulators and all had some difficulties with some aspects of self-care (for example, taking baths) at the time that they were discharged. Ordinarily patients in their condition would not have been allowed to go out to live alone or to live with an aged relative. Other patients in similar condition are usually kept in Farewell Hospital and little or no effort is made to find a place for them. If it had not been for family or friends with a home to offer them, none of these three women would have had a place to go to because the department of welfare would not have maintained their apartments for the length of time that they were in the hospital. Since they did have such a place, they were in a good position to demand release from the hospital when they thought they were ready to go. Thus, the ability to pay one's way in whole or in part (or have someone else pay for one) is a great help in reaching a successful outcome. It not only helps to get out of the hospital, but it may also help to get prosthetic devices or assistive appliances more quickly, to get a more intensive therapy program (for patients who are completely paying their own way), to get better ward service by tipping the help and paying other patients for minor services, and by purchasing certain instruments for passing one's time—e.g., TV set, newspaper subscriptions, books and magazines.

It is clear from what has been said that having an interested family or other outsider is often crucial to success in the program, especially if the patient is mentally, physically, or psychologically unable to be an effective agent for himself. In some cases, family members may become detailed coordinators of the patient's program. They help to keep staff members on their toes by requesting information about the patient's case, by making demands for treatment or other services, by demanding an explanation if service is diminished or information is lacking. They sometimes succeed in keeping a patient on rehab for a longer period of time or getting him back on the program after he has been transferred off. They may provide him with the means of escaping from the hospital when he appears to be stuck there. They may pay for the patient's apartment, for assistive appliances, and for other needs. The patient without outside help and financial resources of his own is at a serious disadvantage, although a few intelligent, aggressive, resourceful persons manage to get quite far without these aids.

We must be careful not to slur over the fact that a patient's physical condition and its improvement or deterioration are of major importance in his success on the rehabilitation program. The most "highly motivated" patient may end up a rehab failure if he has a severe progressive disease which current medicine and therapeutic techniques cannot reverse or overcome in part, as some of the most tragic of our cases testify.

One attribute of success is a good general physical condition aside from the specific disability. In such a case the staff can concentrate on correcting or compensating for the specific disability. The patient can readily take on a relatively vigorous therapeutic program and is likely to be in good enough functional condition to permit a community discharge. The younger amputees are a typical representation of such cases.

Marked improvement in physical function during the course of rehab therapy arouses enthusiasm of the therapeutic staff who will then work harder to bring the case to the most successful possible conclusion and to improve the chances of community placement. Thus, improvement becomes both a cause and a result of more intensive therapy.

Whether or not his physical abilities lead to independence in self-care and locomotion may also be important to a patient's success. If he can do things for himself, he need not depend on the staff for care and thus may be able to get many things done which otherwise are done only haphazardly or not at all. He can get to see people who do not come to him and thus can be more effective as a coordinator of his program than if he is confined to bed or to some wheelchair location where a nurse's aide may happen to put him. The more independent he is, the more he can practice physical skills and thus speed his improvement still further. Thus, again, independence in physical function is both the result and a cause of further progress.

In much the same way the ability to speak is important. The patient who can speak can assert himself, make demands, make his wants known. The more complete aphasic on the rehab program is at a severe handicap and if he does not have some family member working for him, he may well get lost in the shuffle. Of course, the rehab program includes facilities for training in the improvement of speech, but the chances of getting speech therapy—just like the chances of getting any other treatment or service—depend in part on the amount of interest and desire shown and the pressure applied, and it is precisely the patient who is unable to speak who is severely handicapped in expressing his desire and in applying pressure to promote his own cause.

Youth is a favorable attribute regardless of all other characteristics. In fact, patients are often taken on rehab simply because they are young, and the physicians do not want to see these young people dumped on a chronic medical ward with seriously deteriorated old people. Once on rehab, the staff may keep young people who are not making any physical progress and who have no prospect of discharge to the community for much the same reason. Intensive physical therapy is often given to young patients whose prognosis is quite poor. Special programs in group work and other forms of social stimulation are provided for them. Special efforts for placement are made by physicians and social workers in cases that would be abandoned if the patient were older. A whole team meeting may sometimes be taken up in the discussion of one case of a younger person. And such young people are frequently kept on rehab as boarders even after therapy programs have been virtually given up.

THE WAYS OF FAILURE

It is roughly correct to say that the selection for the rehabilitation program itself is blocked if a patient's condition is too good or too poor. That is, if the patient's physical functioning is such that he is completely independent in self-care and ambulation, there is no need seen for a rehab program. On the other hand, if his general physical condition or any particular aspect of it is so severely damaged that the rehabilitation program does not seem likely to result in significant improvement in physical function, he is regarded as a "poor candidate for rehab" and is not likely to be selected. Some patients falling into these categories (mostly the second one) get on the rehab program "by mistake," but are usually eliminated quickly as soon as they are discovered. Thus, these are important characteristics leading to failure.

We may say also that the failure attributes are largely the reverse of the success attributes. Thus passivity and the assumption that one must do no thinking about one's care or treatment or take no initiative to promote one's care and treatment because the staff knows best is likely to lead to one's being forgotten repeatedly or to crucial aspects of one's needs and even of one's prescribed program being neglected or slowed down considerably. "Low motivation" will cause the staff to believe that a patient is not worth working with, getting prosthetic legs for, trying to ambulate, attempting to make a community placement for, and so on. If the patient has no interested family or friends, he is likely to have no place to go to, no one to do favors for him or pay for his needs, no one to put pressure on the staff from the outside. If he is largely physically dependent or mentally incompetent to begin with, the lack of an interested family or friends is almost sure to be fatal to all possibility of success or escape from Farewell Hospital.

So far as physical condition is concerned, complicating disorders which make diagnosis and treatment difficult and prolonged are likely to cause the patient to end up on a nursing unit while still in a poor state of physical function. A very slow response or no response to therapy will discourage the therapists after some months of trying and raise the good possibility of abandonment of the patient. Physical dependence means that others must be relied on for care and this is often not forthcoming. In turn, this may lead to further deterioration or complications. If such physical dependence is combined with extreme passivity and lack of outside interested parties to help the patient, he is likely to receive little attention and become a forgotten man, perhaps hanging around rehab a long time with little result, or perhaps being put off quickly when someone notices him and his unpromising condition. Old age is certainly not an automatic cause for rejection (the bulk of the hospital population is quite advanced in age), but the older person does not have the benefit of the marked bias that the staff shows in favor of youth and is thus more likely to be rejected for other reasons.

In addition to these aspects which are the reverse of the success attributes, we find that those patients who have reputations for being "old bums" with long institutional careers are assumed to be here for the rest of their lives and that not much need be done for them except perhaps to make them a little more independent in self-care so that they will be less of a burden to the custodial staff. Social workers commonly assume that there is no point in making any effort for community placement for such patients, although the patient's reputation can sometimes be overcome with a heroic effort, as in the case of Tom Ormsby.

When there are special difficulties in the care of a patient, the nursing staff is likely to regard him as a poor candidate for rehab. For example, incontinence is often cited as a sign that the patient has been placed on the wrong ward and really should be on a nursing unit, especially if the incontinence continues for more than a few weeks after the patient has arrived on rehab. Some members of the therapeutic staff sometimes question the nursing labels of incontinence and wonder whether it simply means that the patient is not brought a urinal or a bedpan when he or she needs it, but physicians and therapists never spend time on the ward to find out for themselves whether or not this is the case, so they must take the word of the ward nurses. Frequent falls on the part of the patient may also get him classified as an inappropriate rehab candidate and the medical residents are likely to back the nursing staff in this judgment because they are called in to make an examination and write an accident report each time the patient has fallen.

A patient's refusal to help himself when the custodial staff believes he is capable of doing so will also generate pressure to have him removed from rehab. This is particularly true if the patient will not change his view on how independent he should be (for example, continues to call for help and insist that he should be cared for even after weeks of being repeatedly told that his behavior is inappropriate on the rehab unit and he must learn to do things for himself), or if the patient passes his viewpoint on to other patients and thus further subverts the effort to promote self-care on the ward.

Success and failure are the result of an implicit (occasionally explicit) dialogue. Patients have certain (more or less changeable) characteristics. The staff's working definitions of success and failure tend to weed out some, promote others. Patients react to staff actions in ways which enhance their chances of success or failure—sometimes learning the game to some extent and deliberately playing it to get more of what they want. (For example, many patients grasp the notion of "high motivation" and make repeated statements to the staff about how anxious they are to improve their performance and return home.) Staff in turn decide which of the patients' reactions are "realistic" and meaningful in terms of eventual outcome. And so on to a final conclusion when the patient—early or late—is separated from the program.

Institutions for the unwanted

At the time we made our first few visits to the rehabilitation unit at Farewell Hospital a young female patient named Charlene Newcomb was just going through the final stages of arranging discharge from the hospital to her home. She moved around pushing her own wheelchair with assistive devices strapped on to aid her in the movements of her arms and hands. Despite the obvious serious handicap in the use of her body, she seemed to be a remarkably cheerful young woman who had good relationships with many of the other patients as well as with staff members. She was quite happy at the time about the prospect of going home to her husband and baby. She and the therapy staff were convinced that she would be able to perform some of the child-care functions for her baby and thus be an active mother, and also be able to perform some of the lighter housework tasks and thus be a real housewife and not simply a helpless invalid sitting around all day in her apartment.

Charlene Newcomb had come on the rehab unit with such a badly broken body, including spinal cord damage at a high level, that at the time it did not seem likely that she would ever regain any functional use of her extremities or be able to lead any kind of active life again. The period of treatment and retraining was a long one. A number of staff members devoted a great deal of time, effort, and ingenuity to the task of trying to return some useful function to this young woman's limbs. The patient herself was anxious to cooperate and worked hard to achieve this goal. She had something to work for. She had a place to go to, a husband who wanted her back, a baby whom she had scarcely had a chance to begin to rear before her accident. The effort was more successful than anyone at the beginning would have predicted. She left the hospital able to sit up, move around in a wheelchair, do many tasks for herself, for her child, and for her family household.

By the time we started our more systematic observations on the rehab unit Charlene Newcomb was already gone. But we kept hearing about her over and over from some of the older patients and more often from various staff members. Even after we had been there a year, her name kept coming up every now and then, often as a standard of comparison of what the rehabilitation program could do for a patient. After hearing Charlene Newcomb's success story repeatedly throughout our first few months, we began to realize why this was such a notable event worthy of frequent retelling. A dramatic, clear-cut success is rare in this hospital unit. Patients like Charlene Newcomb are not discharged every month. They are not even discharged every year. The New-comb case was a gratifying experience which they cherished particularly because it does not happen very often.

Charlene Newcomb represents a kind of ideal for rehabilitation. She is a patient which rehabilitation as a team of cooperating specialties envisaged in its recent historical development as the kind of patient for whom its services were especially suitable.

This ideal patient is a man or woman in good health—that is, healthy enough for normal physical functioning, preferably a member of a stable family—who is seriously disabled as the result of an accident or sudden illness. A rehabilitation team can then take on the task of correcting the causes of the disability so far as possible, and insofar as the disability cannot be basically corrected, retrain the patient in self-care functions, in ambulation or other means of locomotion, in vocational skills (or perhaps homemaking skills for women), and outfitting the patient with any prosthetic devices or assistive devices which prove useful for increasing the patient's physical capacities. The psychosocial specialties can at the same time help the patient to "accept his disability" and help his or her family through the social and economic crisis that they may face while the patient is hospitalized. Eventually the patient, markedly improved in physical functioning, is brought to the point where he can leave the hospital and return home to the family whose members want him back. If the patient is a man, he returns to work, possibly requiring a change in the type of work and further training before doing so. If the patient is a woman, she returns to her housework and the care of her children, perhaps with some specially devised house arrangements (for example, ramps for wheelchairs or widened doors) and with housekeeping assistance for certain tasks.

Such is the ideal. Such is the kind of patient the rehab program at Farewell Hospital rarely gets. Those with any money or insurance usually stay out of the public hospital system, getting private treatment, conserving their funds by spending much of their time at home while being treated and retrained. The public hospitals get largely poor people with no private physician. The ones who stay in the public system for long treatment or custodial care are those without any interested family or friends, or whose family no longer wants them back or who live in such cramped quarters with such poor facilities for caring for a partly or completely dependent person that the patient's return home would constitute a great burden. They are mostly elderly people past their working years with no dependent children. Some are dependent on welfare aid even before reaching Farewell Hospital and almost all of them are by the time they leave—if they leave.

Even the rehab program, which avoids the most seriously disabled or those who for social reasons seem unlikely to benefit from intensive physical therapy and retraining, gets a population which is far from the staff's ideal. Despite a deliberate bias in favor of youth, most of their patients are elderly. The occupational background of the patients is generally low. A substantial proportion have no family or friends who are interested in them.

For Farewell Hospital as a whole the picture is even more drab. For example, 80 percent of all the patients are above sixty years of age. Many have severe chronic illnesses which are not likely to improve, especially with the minimal medical and nursing care that is given. In many of the cases, the family and friends of these patients cannot even be traced or when traced show no interest in offering them a home. Sixty-three percent of all discharges from this hospital are deaths— that is, almost two-thirds of the admissions live out their lives here.

There are a small number of patients who are injured and disabled in "the prime of life"—the young adult paraplegics and quadriplegics fall into this category. Here it would seem that the rehabilitation program has its ideal. The trouble is that almost all of these patients have been abandoned by their families, if they had one at the time they were disabled. Therefore, there is nowhere to send them when they have reached their "maximum" on the rehab program. The rehabilitation process is truncated and incomplete. The rehab unit ends up being a boarding home for unwanted young men and a severe embarrassment to a staff which prefers to think of its program as a temporary stopover for patients receiving therapy and retraining.

Farewell Hospital is a home for the unwanted. If a patient is wanted, he probably would not have landed in Farewell Hospital in the first place. The minority of wanted patients who come to Farewell for some specific treatment are soon on their way again, usually within a year. The rest—a residue, but a majority residue—languish at Farewell Hospital, and the rehabilitation program gets its share of them.

Even the physical disorders which the physicians and therapists are expected to treat often become secondary. Take, for example, the case of Grant Whitfield, a hemiplegic who spent a few months on the rehab unit before being shunted off to one of the other units in the hospital. Whitfield had been in a general hospital for treatment of his condition and then had been placed on a home-care program. After a short time, his wife complained to the home-care service that she could not take care of her husband at home. She induced the home-care people to hospitalize him, which they did at Farewell Hospital. He was discovered by the rehabilitation director at his weekly selection clinic and moved to the rehabilitation unit. Since he had come to Farewell Hospital from his home, the staff at first had some hope of sending him back to his home when they were through with him. But after the social worker had talked to Whitfield's wife and read the home-care records, it became clear that the wife did not want him back. The wife saw this as a permanent solution to her "problem." At this point the rehabilitation staff threw up its hands, decided that there was no place for him to go to in the community, and after they had decided that he was not receiving any benefit from their program, transferred him to a nursing unit because he was still quite dependent physically.

Rather than say Whitfield is in Farewell Hospital because he is a hemiplegic, it might be more correct to say he is in Farewell Hospital because his wife does not want him at home. Obviously, Farewell Hospital cannot accommodate all the men in the community whose wives do not want them at home. But if the man has a physical disability *and* his wife does not want him, he may very well end up in Farewell as a permanent resident. The physical disability, thus, is often the excuse rather than the reason for hospitalization.

Our data clearly show some of the advantages of having an interested family or friends, especially those who can maintain a home for one or can offer a home when one is ready to leave the hospital. For example, if one has a family who is able to pay for prosthetic devices, he does not have to go through the long waiting period required when prostheses are ordered through the department of welfare. More important still is the fact that having a home available is for many patients crucial to being discharged from the hospital at all.

Our society has many homes for unwanted people. In addition to custodial homes and hospitals like Farewell, we have numerous mental hospitals, institutions for the retarded, nursing homes, old-age homes, training schools for delinquents, and so on. The specific kind of institution a person "qualifies" for is often arbitrary. Many Farewell patients have sufficient signs of mental deterioration or behavior disturbing to others to qualify them for a mental hospital. A few of the patients who were observed, in fact, had been dumped by their families in mental hospitals at an earlier time and some of those now in Farewell eventually end up in nursing homes, old-age homes, or mental hospitals where they will end their lives.

Such institutions all perform much the same function, and we suspect that the choice of which institution the patient goes to is often an accident of the person or agency he happens to fall in the hands of. Thus, a homeless multiple sclerosis patient referred to the city psychiatric unit may be shipped to a state mental hospital, whereas the same person coming into the hands of the rehabilitation medicine unit at the city hospital would be more likely to be shipped to Farewell Hospital for custodial care. To the patient who is stuck in such an institution, it often makes little difference which one he ends up in, except that the facilities and personnel at one may be somewhat more tolerable than those at another.

Although institutions for the unwanted all do much the same thing, they have differing "excuses" for their existence, and these excuses make some difference in how they operate. The active philosophy of a physical rehabilitation unit is the rehabilitation of patients toward greater self-care and, if possible, to return them to the community and even to a job. Much emphasis is placed on physical independence—independence in feeding, dressing, grooming, toileting, locomotion. The cooperative and "motivated" patient is the best bet and receives the most attention. In many mental hospitals there is also an active philosophy of promoting psychological normality—making the patient's behavior more acceptable to the norms of the larger society. Again, the staff tries to promote a form of independence—independence in handling one's daily affairs and being able to relate to others without unusual strain or repeated overt conflict. Again, it is the "motivated" patient who is the most deserving and gets the most attention. Nursing homes and old-age homes occasionally have programs designed to keep inmates active and interested in life. Prisons and training schools sometimes have programs designed to shift the prisoner's way of life to greater conformity with the law-abiding society—providing him with occupational and social skills to live in that society.

But these programs are diluted in a number of ways. For one thing, the inmate must be trained to live in the institution and within a round of life suited to the limitations of the institutional facilities and the convenience of its staff. Sometimes the institutional needs coincide in part with the active therapy or training program. For example, in increasing the patient's ability to care for himself, the training staff is not only increasing the chances of his being discharged from the hospital, but also making the patient less of a bother to the custodial staff if he must stay in the institution. In mental hospitals less bizarre behavior makes a mental hospital an easier place to work in. But often the two aims conflict. In mental hospitals patients are trained for work to maintain the hospital, not for work outside the institution. At Farewell Hospital wheelchairs are well adapted to life within a hospital and the staff is often content to allow patients to remain at this level and not bother to work toward ambulation with or without crutches.

Then, too, if the population is a large one, the active program is likely to involve only a small part of the population. Thus at Farewell, out of almost two thousand beds, only one hundred were devoted to an active rehabilitation program and of these patients about one-third were not on any active program at any given time. Most of the patients entering Farewell Hospital never get into the rehab program at all. Mental hospitals usually have only a few intensive treatment wards and the bulk of the institution is primarily for custodial care. In institutions for the mentally retarded, those defined as "educable" or "trainable" often include only a minority of the total. Rehabilitation programs in prisons and training schools are likely to be for selected prisoners only.

Even those selected for an active program spend only a very small part of their time in the institution receiving therapy or training. It is well known that mental patients on a therapy program commonly get only a few hours of psychotherapy or group therapy each week and perhaps a few more hours of occupational therapy, recreational therapy, and so on. Homes for the aged with recreational programs are likely to have only a few hours a week during regular working

hours when any given patient may actually be participating
in such a program. Likewise, rehab patients spend only a
very small fraction of their time in the treatment programs
which serve as the main justification for maintaining the
rehab unit.

We have also detailed the great lengths of time it takes to
get almost anything done, especially anything which requires
the cooperation of agencies outside of rehab. Patients spend
much of their time just waiting—waiting for admission, for
the various activity programs, for tests, for delivery of appliances, for transfer and discharge. Such delays, too, are typical
in mental hospitals and other institutions for the unwanted,
particularly the large public institutions most unwanted people end up in.

Another characteristic common to such institutions is that
they foster a social and economic dependence. They strip the
patient of all his assets and the possibility of earning any
money. They try to make all his decisions for him and tend
to block independent action whenever it is out of line with
the established practice and policy. Of course, individual staff
members sometimes encourage independent action on the
part of the inmates—for example, suggesting to a patient that
he leave the hospital against advice when the staff is hesitant
about releasing him. But such efforts must be kept under
cover and limited if the staff member does not want to get
into trouble with his superiors and with other public agencies
with whom the hospital must work. Social workers, who like
to think of the institutional inmates as their clients, often find
themselves in a position where they are unable to help the
inmate without subverting the hospital or public agency policies and thus risking their own positions.

For a patient to survive with any possibility of independent
action in such a situation, he must either be able to coordinate
his own program aggressively and skillfully and fight for
action on many aspects of that program, or he must have an
independent agent working on his behalf—an agent who is

independent of the entire institutional system in which he is an inmate. A few patients are able to act fairly effectively as their own agents. A few others have family members or other outsiders who are more or less willing and able to carry out part of this goal—especially offering an escape by providing a place to live. The majority, however, have no such agent and must accept whatever disposition is offered them. They may, for example, accept a foster home placement just to get out of the hospital even though they consider such an arrangement grossly unsatisfactory and hope later to effect a change in their living arrangement. In most cases, they are simply stuck in some part of the hospital with no way of getting out.

Some inmates react to the situation by constructing a tolerably comfortable existence out of their hospital life and reach a point where they no longer want to be dislodged from it. Others submit in conscious defeat and still others continue to struggle for a less restricted life. Many of the aged are so seriously mentally deteriorated that it is a question of whether they can conceive of what is happening to them. Seldom, however, can it be said that the patient selected this form of existence. He fell into it quite by accident so far as he is concerned and the discharges, transfers, and other actions that are taken in his case later on are also largely beyond his control.

A question we might raise is how can an active therapy or rehabilitation program operate in such a setting?

Institutions for the unwanted by definition deal largely with the rejects of our society—the relatively less fit and less appealing members of the human race. In Farewell Hospital, for example, the vast bulk of the population that the rehabilitation program has to select from are "poor candidates for rehab" who must be taken on the program simply because there are no better ones around and because the beds in the rehab unit must be kept 80–90 percent full to justify the existence of the unit. Thus the rehabilitation unit finds itself in much the same position as some public junior colleges who must accept below-average high school graduates and then somehow work with them or devise measures for getting rid of them. Like such colleges, the rehab program is diluted by the necessity of spending much time with clients whom the staff do not consider worth working with. Just as some junior colleges have as their major function convincing the majority of students that they are not college material, the rehab staff has as its major function convincing most patients that they are not rehabilitation material. For patients new to Farewell Hospital, the rehab unit serves more often than not as a means of preparing them for a life in the hospital—as a means of getting the patient to "accept his disability" in a way that was never intended by the social workers who coined this phrase.

By the staff's own working definitions of success and failure, they fail in the majority of cases. Of sixty patients we followed closely through the rehab program at Farewell Hospital, thirty-four were clearly considered failures and another nine showed very slight and dubious improvement. For the staff, rehabilitation is, statistically speaking, a program where failure is the norm, significant improvement and discharge from the hospital an exception, and dramatic success a rarity. In an institutional system which selects the deteriorated, the destitute, the unwanted, and then closes off opportunities for initiative on the part of the inmates, the outcome could scarcely be otherwise.

In other homes for the unwanted, staff members also often experience failure in active therapy and retraining programs. That is one reason why mental hospitals, institutions for the retarded, homes for the aged, and training schools for the delinquent are often considered the backwaters of the health and welfare field and the recruitment of competent personnel is difficult. They commonly have a goal of retraining inmates to a "society" which really does not want them. They work within an institutional setting which stresses a closely regulated life and the suppression of independent judgment by inmates. Thus, such active therapy and rehabilitation programs work in a setting whose requirements are contrary to some of the program's principles.

Most rehabilitation practices, originally designed with the ideal patient in mind, must be adapted to the reality of the actual patient population and the institutional and public agency requirements which control these patients' lives. The care and treatment program must be modified to fit this far-less-than-ideal situation. Soon the staff has difficulty recognizing rehabilitation as they had originally conceived of it. Farewell Hospital, like many similar institutions, has an enormous turnover among its professional staff, many of whom come there right after their formal training program to get a short period of "experience" before moving on to a more agreeable and rewarding position elsewhere. Those staff members who stay around for a number of years come to more or less accept the limited selection of patients, the delays, the institutional assaults upon the patients' initiative, the fact that their program has little relationship to the larger institution where most patients end up feeling rejected and abandoned. It is not surprising, therefore, that most of the more stable professional staff turns its back on the therapy program and spends as much time as possible building professional enclaves of research, administration, and teaching—activity which at least in part serves as an escape from a treatment program which offers little satisfaction and reward.

The stable ongoing part of the rehabilitation unit as well as of the rest of the institution is not the professional therapeutic staff, but the custodial staff. These are the people who keep the institution going day and night, weekends and holidays, hour after hour through the day on the wards. They provide the custodial care which is what most of the inmates are there for anyway. They are the necessary substrata without which the institution could not operate at all.

The professional therapy and placement program, in contrast, touches the lives of only a small minority of the inmates entering the hospital. Although this program is certainly important to some patients who come on the rehab unit, it does not significantly alter the institutional careers of the great majority.

If we look at institutions for the unwanted from a traditional medical and administrative viewpoint, we can often see certain changes which would be helpful to some of the inmates. In Farewell Hospital, for example, there are some patients who can make use of specialized therapy and assistive appliances, and in a small number of cases this may mean the difference between getting out of the hospital and living an independent life outside or spending the rest of one's life in the institution. Providing such services and appliances can certainly be made much more efficient, the periods of waiting can certainly be greatly reduced, the chances of overlooking patients who are in need of special services can be minimized, the financial burden on the patients can be lessened, and patients can be provided with much more information about their case so that they will have a better basis for participating in decisions about their own treatment and disposition, especially about placement in the community. However, even if such reforms are instituted, they would still not deal with some fundamental issues which face the staff.

A central fact to be recognized about an institution such as Farewell Hospital is that it is not so much a hospital in the usual general-hospital sense, but rather is a huge nursing home. Most of the patients who come there do not present medical problems as much as they present problems in providing a viable life for people who have been cast off by the larger society and are too damaged physically, mentally, and socially to re-establish themselves in that society. Treating the institution as if it were primarily a hospital introduces at the outset an obstacle to thinking about how it may be best used to serve the inmates. The same thing may be said about public mental hospitals and about some of the other chronic and custodial institutions which are dominated by medically oriented practices and controlled by medical personnel.*

So long as we have institutions which serve as the dumping ground for our social and medical rejects, we must address ourselves to the question of what we can do for the inmates to make life most livable from the inmates' point of view. Perhaps the first thing the treatment or caretaking staff must do is to become completely aware of the kind of population they have in their institution and to consider what kind of "treatment" or "care" could be considered appropriate for them. Is rehabilitation as traditionally conceived at all suitable for most of these people or is it something that is forced on them like an ill-fitting suit? May the pursuit of physical relearning and independence and return to community life frequently lead the dedicated staff members to give the patient something he cannot use and does not want?

We do not want to imply that the professional rehabilitation staff uncritically practices rehabilitation "by the book." These professional people are aware of the severe physical and social limitations of their patients and the imposed limitations of the institutional structure in which they work. Indeed, they often modify their program to allow for these limitations. But the very fact that they think of their actions as "modifications" points to the root of their major difficulty. The staff commonly sees much of their work as a series of unfortunate, though necessary, compromises that must be made in order to keep the program going. So long as this remains their view of their work and the "material" they have to work with, most of the patients will be defined as "poor candidates for rehabilitation" and most of their efforts will result in failure.

The only way to avoid such failure is to develop different criteria of success. If we were asked: "What changes can we

* See Erving Goffman, "The Medical Model and Mental Hospitalization," in his *Asylums*, pp. 321–386.

make in the rehabilitation program to serve the patients better?" we might reply with the old saw: "If I were you, I wouldn't start from here."

Perhaps such words as "rehabilitation" or "retraining" or "psychotherapy" are stumbling blocks in themselves. They conjure up visions of a group of experts spurring into renewed activity another group of people who have in some way fallen by the wayside of the central stream of life in our society. We may have to shatter such visions if we want to make an effort to see the picture from the viewpoint of the institutional inmate.

We might start by inquiring about the patient: What has this person come to and what does he want to do with what is left of his life? The second part of this question is not easy to answer. You do not find out simply by asking the inmates—not even those who are verbally fluent, and many are not. But much may be accomplished by careful observation of the inmates. What seems to distress them and what seems to satisfy them? Over a period of time patterns of distress and satisfaction can be detected for an individual or even for groups of individuals. Such patterns may then point the way to future activity of the staff with respect to that patient or group of patients.

For many patients, the most important staff activities will be those which make them more comfortable and/or give them something enjoyable to do to occupy their time. In terms of professional specialties, this may mean, for example, that occupational therapy might put less emphasis on functional therapy to promote muscle strength and coordination and self-care skills and more emphasis on a greater variety of "diversionary activities." Group work, in organizing programs and activities, might make the patient's enjoyment the major criterion in selecting things to do, rather than focusing on activities designed to promote social interaction. The ward staff might think less in terms of participating in a medical treatment program and more in terms of providing essential services for the patients' maintenance and comfort. By the way, for this last point we believe that nursing personnel, who are largely trained and committed to medical treatment, are probably not the best suited for such a task—except on units set aside for the treatment of acute illness, post-surgical care, and the like. Untrained persons hired specifically for the job of personal service to patients (including ward housekeeping) would probably satisfy the patient's wants more closely. (Volunteers may do an even better job.)

Given the choice, the patient might—and some of those we observed almost certainly would—choose to spend most of his time sitting or lying around "doing nothing." Such an outcome would be difficult indeed for the ardent rehabilitation specialist to accept. A patient will never learn to care for himself this way and will have no chance of ever escaping some form of custody. Experts in physical medicine can also point out that lack of use leads to atrophy and in extreme cases to regressive changes in body chemistry. But we should keep in mind that "on the average" smokers are much more subject to a number of fatal diseases than non-smokers and gluttons have a shorter life span than those who adhere to a more abstemious diet. Yet in our society, we generally allow people to make a choice on whether or not they want to take these risks. Can we allow the same choice to the aged and disabled, even when they are destitute public charges?

This is not to say that a hospital or a home for the unwanted should be conceived of as simply being allowed to run with no staff input or initiative. The staff can certainly offer inmates much valuable information and advice, and many kinds of treatment and activity. In fact, the more kinds of things the patients are offered, the more choices they will have in constructing the kind of life they want to lead. Thus, variety and diversity of stimuli for the patients might become a goal in itself, with patients being given the choice of whether or not they want to participate. Of course, variety and diversity are difficult to program and that is precisely the reason they are not usually a feature of "total institutions." But again, this is a relative matter, and an increase of diversity in inmate living patterns may be deliberately pursued by a staff which is willing to accept the chance that inmates may make the "wrong" choice.

Appendix A
Data-collection

In the beginning days of the study, the project director (Roth) made a series of preliminary visits to Farewell for the purpose of meeting staff members and becoming familiar with the physical setting. Six weeks after his arrival, he was joined by the assistant project director (Eddy). For the next four months, we spent several days each week becoming familiar with the work of the rehab unit and the institution within which it was located. We made it a point to be present not only when the regular therapeutic staff was on duty, but also on days and during hours when members of the rehab team were off duty. During these months, an effort was made to learn as much as possible about the treatment and management setting in which patients found themselves as participants in the life and activities of the rehab unit.

Information was obtained by reading staff memoranda and reports in which patients were evaluated, observing therapeutic sessions and formal meetings in which patients were discussed, discussing treatment and management activities and decisions with staff members so as to learn the rationale behind these, interviewing and observing a small group of new patients on the ward so as to ascertain some of the events in which patients became involved, and attending formal ward programs so that all the patients would come to know us.

From the beginning, a record of observations and interviews made in the field was kept. Following each field experience, field notes were dictated and subsequently transcribed by a secretary who had no connection with the hospital or anyone in it.

After five months of preliminary observations, plans were made for a more systematic and intensive approach to the research. During the initial phase, it had become clear that it would not be feasible to have large numbers of patients fill out paper and pencil questionnaires. A high proportion of patients had disabilities rendering reading or writing difficult or impossible; others had only a limited command of English. Any instruments of this nature would have to be filled out by the researchers themselves. One form was developed to guide the accumulation of background data for each patient.

At this time the more general questions of the study were formulated and translated into a framework of more specific questions under topical headings. This outline served as a guide to the type of research information to be collected on each patient as well as a means of indexing field-note material. This ensured a more adequate collection of comparable data for each patient as well as providing a means for the classification of interviews, hospital reports, and observations.

Three ways of indexing field notes were developed. The first, as described above, was a content index; the second was a name index; and the third was an index used for the purpose of indicating material pertaining to different types of formal meetings or specialty groups. After the field notes had been transcribed, both of us read them and classified their contents. Project secretaries kept files of index cards on which were recorded all the page entries on which a particular topic appeared, a name of a staff member or patient was mentioned, or a formal meeting or specialty group was discussed. By using these indexes we were able to find all the material on a given topic, person, or formal group.

At this point the more intensive collection of data on the careers of patients on the rehab wards began. Four part-time research assistants joined us. These were all male graduate students in anthropology, sociology, or social psychology. Three were American-born and one was a native of Trinidad of Chinese ancestry. Of the three native Americans, one spoke Spanish fluently and had done anthropological field work in Guatemala. This student was particularly helpful in communicating with the Spanish-speaking patients and staff members (although he did much else, too).

Each of the sixty patients who were admitted to the rehabilitation wards during a five-month period was assigned to one of the six researchers. The field worker was then responsible for interviewing and observing the patient from his arrival on the ward (or even before, in the case of patients who came to rehab from other wards within Farewell) until his discharge. If the patient was discharged within Farewell, he was interviewed once or twice following his transfer. Attempts were made to observe the patient in the formal therapeutic program, on the ward, and any other areas where he could be found. All official meetings at which a patient was discussed were attended, and the staff responsible for his care were interviewed and observed in their interactions with the patient.

We purposely selected all the patients who entered the ward during a given period of time so as to get as full an idea as possible of what happened to a great variety of patients. Even though one of our patients was only on the ward for approximately five hours and a few others were there only a matter of days, we continued to include them as examples of types of things that happen to some patients.

By following closely the career patterns of sixty patients, we inevitably attended nearly all formal meetings concerned with patient care for a period of a year, and many meetings for the following six months. We soon learned that the formal scheduling of patients for certain meetings did not necessarily mean that they would be discussed. The fact that we were actually present ourselves and therefore not reliant on official records provided us with many opportunities to keep note of decisions and discussions about patients and to observe the later developments which might influence these.

In addition to observing the formal meetings, we spent considerable time in the therapy areas of physical and occupational therapy. Professional norms about confidentiality prevented our observation of the patient during social work interviews and psychological testing. Insofar as possible, however, we observed the patient at work and could see for ourselves his progress or lack of progress and how the staff interacted with him.

A great deal of time was also spent on the wards, and we soon became known to most of the patients who were around during the intensive period of our study and thus expanded our data to include material on more than our sixty cases. Although some patients tended to view us as physicians (in the case of the male researchers) or a social worker (in the case of the female researcher), most gradually realized we were neither of these, and they seemed to accept our role as persons who could not help them in any substantial way (we did occasionally bring them items from the store, write letters, and on rare occasions made minor interventions with the staff on their behalf), but who were interested in them and what they thought. In the initial stages some patients suspected us of being investigators from the department of welfare or the department of hospitals, but the fact that we were around in the evenings, early morning, weekends, and holidays gradually convinced them (we hope) that we could not possibly have anything to do with the usual staff. Also, of course, we tried to exercise great care so that whatever a patient told us was treated with confidentiality.

We do not mean to imply that all patients freely trusted us or talked freely with us. Some patients were aphasics or otherwise too ill to communicate with anyone. A few preferred to have as little to do with us as possible. On the whole, however, most seemed glad to talk with us. Again, the fact that we were around so much meant that we did not have to rely solely on talking with patients, but had many opportunities to observe even the very ill or uncommunicative. We also found that sometimes one of us could relate effectively to a patient where another one of us was unable to. In such a case, we did not hesitate to redistribute our "case loads" to take advantage of the opportunity.

During a three- to four-month period in the middle of our intensive period of field work (right after the intake of our sixty cases had been completed), we carried out two special observational projects whose results are presented in this book.

One of these was a record of the activity engaged in by each patient and the place where he was located at a given time of day. We did not follow any one patient throughout the day. Rather, we relied on two kinds of surveys. One consisted of an observer stationing himself in one of the several areas where rehab patients congregated (cubicle area, dayroom, hallway on rehab floor, the several therapy rooms) and recording the activities of all patients present. (This included records of time spent in various activities in the PT gyms and the OT shops which we draw upon in parts of Chapter 6.)

The other was a series of rounds of all hospital areas (including the grounds) where we knew rehab patients sometimes went and recording the location and activity of the rehab patients observed. (In each round, there were always a few who eluded us, but they were not always the same ones.) On a given patient we have a record of his activity for different times of the day on different days beginning with the time patients get up in the morning to the time when the late TV watchers go to bed at night. By combining a series of such observations we can construct a "typical day" which does not represent any specific day of observation, but does represent a distribution of the patient's time and activities.

The data-collection for the second special project sometimes was carried on simultaneously with the first, sometimes separately, depending on how difficult the particular task of recording proved to be. This project consisted of obtaining information on the following:

1. Records of "who talks to whom" in given areas for periods of one to two hours in specific locations—e.g., day room, male ward, female ward.

2. Running census of rehab patients at a given time over the entire hospital, their location, whether they were alone or with someone, and if the latter, with whom.

Records 1 and 2 were made during the same three- to four-month period mentioned above. The periods of observation were varied so the entire day from 6:00 A.M. to 11:00 P.M. was covered.

3. Our field notes for the entire period of observation were examined for indications of groupings of patients.

The tabulations from 1 and 2 were combined and quantity of interaction between patients was arbitrarily divided into three levels—high, middle, low. Field-note information was used to make decisions in doubtful cases.

Note that the "interaction patterns" constructed from these observations represent interactional groupings rather than common characteristics or reputation. True, members of a given group may share important attributes, but we did not group them together for that reason. The women we placed in the alcoholic group have a staff reputation of being alcoholics (and thus gave us a convenient label), but we placed them in the same group because they frequently hung out together and interacted relatively less with other patients. There were two other women who were labeled alcoholics by the staff, but we did not place them in this group because they had little or nothing to do with any of the alcoholic group members.

The most intensive phase of our research lasted about one year. At the end of this year, the four research assistants had left the staff. However, since several of our patients had not yet been discharged from the ward, we continued to visit the hospital regularly for two or three days each week. There was a gradual decrease in these visits as fewer of our sample of patients remained on the ward and as the need became greater for more time to devote to the analysis of our material. Toward the end of the study, visits were made only once every month or six weeks, and were largely confined to trying to find out what had happened to the four or five patients who were still on the rehab service.

In one sense, the research approach employed in this study involved a continual analysis of data. The persistent longitudinal observation of persons and events led to the development of hypotheses as further observations were made. Observed regularities in human behavior led to predictions about what would happen and the testing of these predictions against the social fact of what actually did happen.*

In addition to this type of analysis which occurred in the field, however, other types of analyses were undertaken upon the completion of field work. Case summaries were prepared

---

* Howard S. Becker, "Problems of Inference and Proof in Participant Observation," *American Sociological Review*, vol. 23 (December, 1958), pp. 652–660.

for each of the sixty patients which presented, in an abbreviated form, their social characteristics, the timing of events they experienced while on the wards, the official services rendered to them by the staff, staff evaluations made of them at different points in their career, their relationships to other patients, family, and friends, their conceptions of rehabilitation and the outcome of their case with respect to discharge from the ward. These summaries were useful for checking and documenting generalizations about various aspects of patients' care on rehab. In the same way, summary statements constructed with the help of our index about the work of given specialties, the decision-making in team meetings, the ward routines, the off-rehab life, and the many other subjects which fell into the purview of our observations were used in producing our description of the rehab program and the career of the patients who passed through it.

Appendix B
Some disability and social
characteristics of the sample
group of sixty patients

AGE, SEX, AND DISABILITIES

Disability	Under 40		40–49		50–59		60–69		70–79		80 plus		Total	
	M	F	M	F	M	F	M	F	M	F	M	F	M	F
Arthritis	—	—	—	—	1	—	1	—	—	—	—	—	2	—
Alcoholic poly-neuritis	—	—	—	1	—	—	1	2	—	—	—	—	1	3
Amputee	—	—	2	—	3	1	1	2	1	—	—	—	7	3
Cerebral palsy	—	1	—	—	—	—	—	—	—	—	—	—	—	1
Fracture	—	—	—	—	—	1	—	1	1	3	—	—	1	5
Hemiplegia:														
Left	—	1	2	—	—	1	2	1	—	4	—	—	4	5
Right	—	2	1	1	3	2	2	1	2	1	1	—	9	5
Multiple sclerosis	—	—	1	1	1	2	—	—	—	—	—	—	2	5
Parkinson's disease	—	—	—	—	—	—	—	—	1	—	—	—	—	1
Spinal cord	2	—	—	—	1	—	1	—	—	1	—	—	3	1
Miscellaneous	—	—	—	—	1	—	1	—	—	1	—	—	2	1
Total cases	2	4	6	2	9	7	8	7	5	9	1	—	31	29

RELIGIOUS AFFILIATION AND ETHNIC BACKGROUND

Place of Birth, Race and Sex	Religious Affiliation				
	Protestant*	Catholic	Jewish	Unknown	Total
Continental U.S.					
White: M	—	3	1	—	4
F	5	7	2	—	14
Negro: M	12	—	—	—	12
F	6	—	—	1	7
Puerto Rico					
White: M	—	1	—	—	1
Virgin Islands					
Negro: M	1	—	—	1	2
F	—	1	—	—	1
West Indies					
Negro: M	4	1	—	—	5
F	1	—	—	—	1
White: F	1	—	—	—	1
Canada:					
White: F	1	—	—	—	1
Europe:					
White: M	1	4	2	—	7
F	2	1	1	—	4
Total cases	34	18	6	2	60

* Includes two Greek Orthodox.

OCCUPATION IN PERCENT

Occupation	Male	Female	Total Sample
Professional	6.5	3.4	5.0
Small business	9.6	—	5.0
Clerical, sales	6.5	37.9	21.7
Semi- or unskilled	71.0	48.4	60.0
None	3.2	6.9	5.0
Unknown	3.2	3.4	3.3
Total	100.0	100.0	100.0
Total cases	31	29	60

MARITAL STATUS (in Percent)

Marital Status	Male	Female	Total Sample
Married	48.4	17.2	33.3
Separated or divorced	19.3	20.7	20.0
Widowed	9.7	34.5	21.7
Single	22.6	27.6	25.0
Total	100.0	100.0	100.0
Total cases	31	29	60

Appendix C
Characteristics of interaction group members

Groups and Number of Members*	Sex, Age, and Ethnic Characteristics	Social Class Reputation	Condition
Respectable Women 7 central and 1 peripheral; 3 central members are "stars" in that they are involved in most of the interaction within the group and have many connections with patients outside the group.	Female; 50 to 75 years; White; Protestant and Catholic.	All of middle-class or upper lower-class background in terms of occupations, home ownership, area of residence, etc. Considered good respectable women by staff, even though staff members are sometimes annoyed by some of their demands.	All mentally intact and alert. All are mobile, mostly via wheelchair.
Jewish Group 4 central and 4 peripheral.	Central: 3 males, 1 female. Peripheral: 4 females; 42 to 63 years for central members, 1 of peripheral is 90, 1 is 26; White; Jewish (it is not clear whether the fact that they are all Jewish is incidental to their interaction or is a central aspect of it).	All the central members have solidly middle-class backgrounds, as do 3 of the peripheral members; 1 of the peripheral members has a lower-class immigrant background and seems to be partly accepted by some of the others more out of sympathy than anything else.	All are mentally intact and alert except for one of the peripheral members who is sometimes considered crazy because of her insistent complaints. All are mobile in the wheelchair and in 1 case ambulatory. Considered by the rehab staff as good rehabilitation candidates although 1 of the central members is eventually suspected of having a severe psychological difficulty because they cannot get rid of him.

*The group labels are our own, although "young adult" is in common use among staff and patients, and "alcoholics" is sometimes used by staff.

Alcoholics 5 central and 1 peripheral.	Female; 46 to ? years; all Negroes except Brant; Protestant.	All of lower-class background. All of the central members are regarded by the staff as alcoholics and often are described by nursing staff as vulgar and abusive.	They are generally regarded as mentally subnormal or deteriorated, especially Truman, Brant, and Parkill.
Young Adults 11 central and 4 peripheral (all of these were never together at the same time, and 2 among the earliest to go had been gone some time before 2 of the latest ones arrived).	All the central members are male, as are the 2 older peripheral members. 1 peripheral member is a girl in her early 20s, 1 a woman in her early 30s; central members are all in their late teens or 20s, 2 peripheral members are young women and 2 others are men—1 in his 50s and 1 in his 60s; White, Negro, and Puerto Rican; Protestant and Catholic (race and religion are probably incidental in this group with age and sex being the predominant selective factors).	Largely lower class. Most of these men were disabled before they became involved in any occupations. There are two important exceptions, Lombardi and Streich, whose family class position would seem to be quite definitely middle class in the occupational structure. It should be noted too that the 2 Puerto Rican members, although from lower-class backgrounds, have strongly interested families who do eventually take them home.	All are regarded as mentally intact and alert. Of the 11 central members, 9 are paraplegics or quadriplegics and 2 have muscular dystrophy. They vary in mobility from James, who in his wheelchair is by far the most mobile patient on the rehab unit, to Ashby, who has almost no use of his extremities at all and is completely dependent for almost all his personal needs on the staff or other patients.

Groups and Number of Members	Sex, Age, and Ethnic Characteristics	Social Class Reputation	Condition
Old Timers 4 central and 1 peripheral; Marsh and Kent are the main axis of this group; 1 of the central group is not on rehab at the moment, but is a rehab alumnus who spends a great deal of her time on the rehab unit.	Female; 30 to 55 years; Negro; Protestant.	All have occupational backgrounds as domestics or similar level of work, but their personal interaction pattern (and many other aspects of their relationship to the rehab unit) differs sharply from that of the domestic group described. Also, all the central members have been in the hospital for 4 years or more, mostly on the rehab unit. The peripheral member is a relative newcomer.	All are mentally intact and alert. The 3 central members now on the rehab unit are all paraplegics or quadriplegics of limited mobility. (Kent's mobility increased considerably after she received her electric wheelchair.) The rehab alumnus, an amputee, is highly mobile in a wheelchair and therefore comes to see her old friends.
Domestics Very loose group of 7 or 8 women. Gump, the most central member, has some rather strong connections with people outside of this group, especially with 3 members of the respectable women's group.	Female; late-50s to mid-70s; Negro; Protestant	All worked as domestics or in servant-type work (e.g., restroom attendant) or low-level unskilled laborer (laundress). They have no particularly good or bad reputation among the staff and largely go unnoticed.	The group includes 1 aphasic who later became able to communicate to a limited extent. None of the others are regarded as seriously mentally subnormal or deteriorated. All can move about, usually in a wheelchair, but some have great difficulty with the wheelchair and therefore do not move about a good deal.

Newcomers

A very loose group of 8 or perhaps two groups of 4 each with a slight connection between them. Since they were newcomers whom we observed for only a few months when we were slacking off on our observations, we are much less certain of the development of this group than of the others so far discussed. They were perhaps thrown together because they *were* new (it is interesting that the two groups of 4 each represent two levels of newness—the more solid group of 4 having come in within a fairly short period of time during the summer and the looser group of 4 having come in somewhat later within a very short span of time), and possessed some rather obvious common characteristics of age, sex, and race.

Female; 50s to 80s; White

All considered mentally intact. All are wheelchair bound but can get around by themselves. But most of them are very slow in a wheelchair and therefore their range of movement is not wide.

Groups and Number of Members	Sex, Age, and Ethnic Characteristics	Social Class Reputation	Condition
Italian 4 central and 1 peripheral; the main interaction here is the Di-Cresce–Mercuri pair, with Tasso and DiCostanzo and to a lesser extent Brazzi being taken into their orbit occasionally because of the common language. In fact, all the central members of this group are individuals who were near-isolates before they discovered one another's common language and background.	2 females and 2 males among central members, peripheral member is male; mid-50s to early 70s; White—all Italian; Catholic.	All of lower-class background with limited education.	The 2 women and the peripheral male considered somewhat mentally deteriorated. The men are fairly mobile in a wheelchair, the women only slightly so.
X Group (for want of a name) 4 members; Brodsky is the person who serves as the hub of the group.	2 males and 2 females; 40s to 60s; White; all Catholic except 1 who is Jewish (religion in this case seems to be incidental).	Wide range of educational and occupational background from 1 member with several years of college education and a former technical occupation to another who is regarded as having been an unemployed bum. (It is these 2 in fact who have by far the closest association within the group.)	One member is aphasic and it is unusual for aphasic patients to be brought out of isolation even to the limited degree that she is here. The other 3 members are all considered mentally intact and 1 of them is regarded as highly intelligent though his voice is extremely weak and he has difficulty expressing himself. Physically, 1 is almost helpless and relies on another one who is normally mobile and ambu-

The Sitters 3 men who seem to have difficulty understanding one another, but still spend much time with each other, often just sitting side by side for long periods. They often kid one another, but the meaning of their remarks was usually incomprehensible to the observer.	Male; 60s and 70s; Negro—2 from the British West Indies; Protestant.	Lower class, but with steady jobs—definitely not bums.	All had CVAs with serious hemiplegia, 2 of them partly aphasic but with considerable recovery.
Spanish 3 men who are very loosely connected. The looseness of the connection is due mainly to the fact that 2 of them have important associations with people in other parts of the hospital and the third one receives many visits from his family. Apparently brought together in a limited way by their common language, and in the case of 2 of them, by a common disability.	Male; 50s and 60s; White—2 Puerto Rican and 1 European background; Catholic.	All in good trades with steady work and income.	2 were bilateral amputees and 1 a hemiplegic who learned to walk. All were mentally intact except that José had some aphasia in the beginning from which he was making a good recovery.

Selected references

Barney G. Glaser and Anselm L. Strauss. *Awareness of Dying*. Chicago: Aldine Publishing Company, 1965.
Uses a scheme of "awareness contexts" to classify the nature of information manipulation among hospital staff, patient, and his family. The scheme is applicable to the manipulation of information other than dying in a variety of service institutions.

Erving Goffman. *Asylums*. Garden City, N.Y.: Doubleday Anchor Book, 1961.
Four essays on institutions for the "mentally ill." The essays deal with the organized structure of the institutions, the career of patients, the "underlife" of patients, and the relationship of psychiatry to institutional operations.

Jules Henry. *Culture Against Man.* New York: Random House Vintage Edition, 1965.
A graphic account of the patterns of life forced on the socially weak in our society. Psychoanalytic interpretations are often applied.

Howard R. Kelman, "An Experiment in the Rehabilitation of Nursing Home Patients," *Public Health Reports,* 77 (April 1962), 356–366.
A report on an experiment which indicates that the addition of rehabilitation services makes no measurable difference in the lives of nursing home patients.

Elliott A. Krause. "After the Rehabilitation Center," *Social Problems,* 14 (Fall 1966), 197–206.
This paper deals with the evaluation and disposition of non-institutionalized severely disabled persons. It examines the manner in which organizational and societal demands and definitions of success determine the decisions which counselors and other professionals make about their disabled clients.

Marjorie Fiske Lowenthal. *Lives in Distress.* New York: Basic Books, 1964.
Details the paths to another kind of institution for the un-wanted—the mental hospital.

Thomas Mathiesen. *The Strategies of the Weak.* Oslo: Institute for Social Research, 1962.
A study of a cross between a prison and mental hospital in Norway. Particular attention is given to the manner in which the inmates try to overcome their organizationally weak bargaining position.

Martin Rein. "The Social Service Crisis," *Trans-Action,* 1 (May 1964), 3–6, 31–32.
Describes the process of "creaming" by service agencies which quite consistently concentrate their services on the best prospects for success and tend to ignore those most in need of the services. Directly applicable to most rehabilitation services.

Anselm Strauss, Leonard Schatzman, Rue Bucher, Danuta Ehrlich, and Melvin Sabshin. *Psychiatric Ideologies and Institutions.* New York: The Free Press, 1964.
A major theme of this book is that the nature of treatment of patients is determined more by the ideology of the staff than by

available treatment technologies, a point applicable to other institutions—including chronic disease hospitals—committed to a "mental health" approach. See especially Parts 3, 4, and 5.

Marvin B. Sussman, ed. *Sociology and Rehabilitation.* Washington, D.C.: American Sociological Association, no date.
A series of papers prepared for a conference on "Sociological Theory, Research and Rehabilitation." Includes papers on historical background, conceptual discussions of the rehabilitation process, and summary reports of selected research in the sociology of rehabilitation.

Peter Townsend. *The Last Refuge.* London: Routledge & Kegan Paul, 1962.
An intensive survey of the provision made for the unwanted aged in England and Wales.

For Product Safety Concerns and Information please contact our
EU representative GPSR@taylorandfrancis.com Taylor & Francis
Verlag GmbH, Kaufingerstraße 24, 80331 München, Germany